Oklahoma Notes

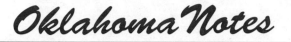

Clinical Sciences Review for Medical Licensure
Developed at
The University of Oklahoma College of Medicine

Ronald S. Krug, *Series Editor*

Suitable Reviews for:
United States Medical Licensing Examination (USMLE), Step 2
Federation Licensing Examination (FLEX)

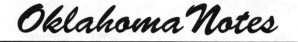

Oklahoma Notes

Psychiatry

L. Blaine Shaffer
Ronald S. Krug

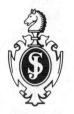

Springer-Verlag
New York Berlin Heidelberg London Paris
Tokyo Hong Kong Barcelona Budapest

L. Blaine Shaffer, M.D.
Department of Psychiatry
College of Medicine
The University of Oklahoma
2808 South Sheridan Road
Tulsa, OK 74129
USA

Ronald S. Krug, Ph.D.
Department of Psychiatry and
  Behavioral Sciences
Health Sciences Center
The University of Oklahoma
Oklahoma City, OK 73190
USA

Library of Congress Cataloging-in-Publication Data
Shaffer, Blaine.
    Psychiatry / Blaine Shaffer, Ronald Krug.
      p.   cm. — (Oklahoma notes)
    ISBN 0-387-97957-3. — ISBN 3-540-97957-3
    1. Psychiatry—Outlines, syllabi, etc.   I. Krug Ronald S.
  II. Title. III. Series.
    [DNLM: 1. Mental Disorders—outlines. WM 18 S525p]
  RC457.2S43   1993
  616.89—dc20
  DNLM/DLC
  for Library of Congress   92-48924
                                   CIP

Printed on acid-free paper.

Production managed by Jim Harbison; manufacturing supervised by Jacqui Ashri.
Camera-ready copy prepared by the authors.
Printed and bound by Edwards Brothers, Inc., Ann Arbor, MI.
Printed in the United States of America.

9 8 7 6 5 4 3

ISBN 0-387-97957-3 Springer-Verlag New York Berlin Heidelberg
ISBN 3-540-97957-3 Springer-Verlag Berlin Heidelberg New York

Preface to the
Oklahoma Notes

In 1973 the University of Oklahoma College of Medicine instituted a requirement for passage of the Part 1 National Boards for promotion to the third year. To assist students in preparation for this examination a two-week review of the basic sciences was added to the Curriculum in 1975. Ten review texts were written by the faculty. In 1987 these basic science review texts were published as the *Oklahoma Notes* ("Okie Notes") and made available to all students of medicine who were preparing for comprehensive examinations. Over a quarter of a million of these texts have been sold nationally. Their clear, concise outline format has been found to be extremely useful by students preparing themselves for nationally standardized examinations.

Over the past few years numerous inquiries have been made regarding the availability of a Clinical Years series of "Okie Notes." Because of the obvious utility of the basic sciences books, faculty associated with the University of Oklahoma College of Medicine have developed texts in five specialty areas: Medicine, Neurology, Pediatrics, Psychiatry, and Surgery. Each of these texts follows the same condensed outline format as the basic science texts. The faculty who have prepared these texts are clinical educators and therefore the material incorporated in these texts has been validated in the classroom.

Each author has endeavored to distill the "need to know" material from their field of expertise. While preparing these texts, the target audience has always been the clinical years student who is preparing for Step 2 examinations.

A great deal of effort has gone into these texts. I hope they are helpful to you in studying for your licensure examinations.

Ronald S. Krug, Ph.D.
Series Editor

Preface

We have arranged this review text in an order that makes clinical sense. We have assumed that the student has had considerable experience with the field of Psychiatry via didactic courses, clinical rotations or both. The first chapter is an Introduction to Psychiatry with significant persons and events in the growth of the field being noted. Chapter 2 focuses on general diagnostic categories and the major intervention strategies that are used in the field. Chapter 3 presents patient management in detail so that in the later chapters, as disorders are being presented, the student can have the management strategies clearly in mind.

Chapters 4 through 12 review each of the major psychiatric disorders in detail and provide suggestions regarding the etiology and appropriate treatment of the disorder. Chapter 13 focuses on the special problems of children. That is, while children can have most of the same disorders as can adults, there are disorders that are diagnosed in childhood that are different from those of adults.

Chapter 14 focuses on special issues in the practice of psychiatry such as sleep issues, forensic psychiatry, AIDS, etc. Chapter 15 is devoted to psychiatric emergencies in both adults and children.

This is a review text and should not be substituted for more complete texts. The authors do not recommend that this book be used as a course text except in those academic offerings that are specifically directed to an overview of psychiatry.

To use this review text effectively, the beginning student should start with the first chapter and progress through the text in a systematic fashion. This recommendation is based on the fact that subsequent chapters may reference material in earlier chapters and, if the student is skipping around, the building on one chapter by another may be short-circuited.

The authors believe this text would be helpful in preparation for the various licensing/certification examinations, including Step 2 of the United States Medical Licensure Examinations (USMLE), Medical Sciences Knowledge Profile (MSKP), and the Foreign Medical Graduate Examination in the Medical Sciences (FMGEMS).

The authors wish to gratefully acknowledge the efforts of Ms. Susan Jordan and Ms. Peggy Shaffer for their invaluable assistance in the preparation of the manuscript.

Good luck to you in your studies.

L. Blaine Shaffer
Ronald S. Krug

Contents

CHAPTER 1

INTRODUCTION

I. **INTRODUCTION**

    A. <u>Psychiatry</u> is the medical specialty which has grown out of the management of persons who are demonstrating behaviors, reflective of the "mind", which are deemed "abnormal". The word behavior is employed as a general term to include thoughts, acts, verbalizations, perceptions, emotions, etc..

    B. <u>Definitions of Abnormal</u>: very tightly tied to philosophic concepts and ethics.

        1. Statistical definitions of abnormality reflect the Consequentialist philosophical stance of "the greatest good for the greatest number of persons." Applied here, whatever the majority behavior is, is defined as normal. Deviations from the norm are considered to be abnormal.

        2. Absolutely pathological behavior follows from the Deontologist philosophical stance that some things are in and of themselves either right or wrong, or good or bad. In looking at pathologic behaviors, some behaviors are judged abnormal regardless of the number of persons who manifest the behavior; e.g., hallucinations.

        3. From a psychiatric standpoint it is more productive to view behaviors as adaptive versus maladaptive without a judgement of right or wrong.

    C. It is significant that American Psychiatry does not recognize political difference as being a mental illness. This is in opposition to some other countries where persons who hold different political ideas and beliefs are often sequestered in institutions designed for persons with mental disorders.

II. **ASSUMPTIONS AND RATIONALE REGARDING MENTAL DISORDERS**

    Conflicts in living are similar and occur for all persons. The manner in which the conflicts are handled makes the difference between whether one is "normal," psychotic, neurotic, a personality disorder, a psychophysiologic converter, an adjustment disorder, etc. <u>I.e., humans differ regarding their defense mechanisms for handling conflict.</u> That difference may be genetic, inherited, learned, cultural, etc.

    A. Persons with <u>psychotic symptoms</u> have <u>few effective defense mechanisms</u> to deal with conflicts. Probably anyone can be made acutely psychotic by increasing conflict to the point that coping strategies normally used cannot handle the associated affect.

B. Persons with <u>anxiety, dissociative, or psychosomatic symptoms</u> handle conflicts with defense mechanisms at an unconscious level. Their symptoms are a combination of the underlying impulse and the defense mechanism. Symptoms are <u>EGO DYSTONIC</u>; they bother the person.

C. Persons with <u>personality disorders</u> handle conflicts with <u>life-long maladaptive behavior patterns</u>. Their behaviors bother other persons not them. They are <u>EGO SYNTONIC</u> for the patient.

III. GENERAL ETIOLOGIES AND THEORIES

A. The "mind" is a concept which creates problems when we try to understand people who are manifesting behaviors that are maladaptive.

1. The human being is a biological system. The organ of the mind is the brain. The process of the brain is the mind.

2. If we focus on a single neuron or sets of neurons and their functioning, the concept of "mind" gets blurred.

3. If we focus on the concept of "mind", then neuronal functions become an inadequate concept and get blurred.

4. Man's ability to **SYMBOLIZE** is what elevates him above the simple stimulus response of a biologic system. This symbolization is often what is deemed to be "abnormal" or maladaptive.

B. The "Mind-Body" split: A concept rooted in religious thought.

1. Mind is the seat of the soul
2. The soul cannot be sick
3. Therefore the mind is not a part of the body which can be ill.

C. "<u>Bio-psycho-social</u>" assumptions

1. **Host:** the individual who is the focus of attention.

2. **Agent:** the causative/etiologic entity which is introduced to the host.

3. **Environment:** the surrounding in which the host and the agent are located.

4. The assumption is that the Host, Agent and Environment interact together to produce the observed maladaptive behavior.

5. This formula is central, for example, to the concept of addictions being a disease. E.g., a host (often with a genetic predisposition); ingests a drug (which has addicting properties); in an environment that supports and encourages the use of the agent, or has produced the stress that has made the drug effect attractive. Over time this results in the disease of chemical dependence.

   Also, it is central in understanding the course of mental disorder. E.g., a host who has a genetic predisposition to Schizophrenia, may be stabilized with a given medication. However, they may be "discharged" from a protective environment of a psychiatric hospital into a "homeless" environment which then destabilizes the person.

D. Neurobiologic Considerations

1. **Anatomic sites**

   a. Cortex: the portion of the brain that is responsible for symbolic functioning of different types.

      The neocortex receives data from the external world through sense organs. Perception is in the neocortex. However, perceptions lack emotional coloring without the limbic system.

   b. Subcortex: controls the automatic and more vegetative/primitive functioning of the organism.

      (1) **Limbic System:** The limbic system is comprised of the phylogenetically old cortex and its associated structures; the hippocampus, fornix, mammillary bodies, anterior thalamic nuclei, cingulate gyrus, septal nuclei and amygdala.

      This system is arranged into circuits and influences behavioral expression regulated by the hypothalamus.

      The functional regulative activities of the limbic system include: modulation and coordination of the central processes of emotional elaboration; motivation; establishment of conditioned reflexes; and memory storage.

      There are rich connections between limbic system and neocortex. The frontal lobes are the major neocortical representatives of the limbic system. They monitor and modulate limbic mechanisms. E.g., the Prefrontal and Frontal areas of the brain have been significantly implicated in "socially appropriate behavior"; and consequently, when disorders are seen which include social inappropriateness in their syndrome, the Frontal areas and correlated limbic system are implicated.

Behaviors associated with the limbic system:

There is a satiety center whose destruction leads to hyperphagia;

Lesions of the ventral-medial nucleus of the hypothalamus results in overeating and obesity.

There is apparently a thirst center; destruction leads to loss of the urge to drink fluids.

Kluver-Bucy Syndrome: first established in monkeys. After removal of the temporal lobe and amygdala, hyperaggressive animals became tame and submissive. Also displayed visual agnosia, a tendency to oral exploration, and hypersexuality.

Stimulation of the septal brain area has demonstrated a pleasure or reward center.

(2) Reticular Activating System (RAS)

The brainstem reticular formation consists of a network of nerve cells located in the lower brainstem at a point where all sensory and motor impulses pass on the way in and out of the brain.

The RAS alerts the brain to wakefulness so it can deal with stimuli.

The RAS **facilitates and inhibits** a great range of data.

The RAS influences excitability of afferent relays in the spinal cord thus influencing voluntary and involuntary motor performance.

The orienting response. RAS modulates and inhibits transmission of impulses peripherally or at the first central synapse of the major afferent pathways. Thus it functions as a selective filter of incoming information; e.g., during attention focusing, the RAS may exclude irrelevant sensory input.

Psychotic behaviors. Research has associated dysfunction of the RAS with schizophrenia. It is proposed that lesions of the RAS have a wider effect than do lesions elsewhere, since they involve the filter system through which the entire CNS is alerted to the task of integrating activity.

Other data associating psychotic-like behavior with RAS include the fact that drugs which control psychoses are effective in the limbic system and reticular formation. They work in the synaptic cleft but do not penetrate the neuron. In the cleft they affect neuro-transmitters.

c. Interaction: Some processes (e.g., memory) represent an interaction between the Cortical and Subcortical areas.

2. **Neurotransmitters:** In the last few decades much focus has been on the issue of "chemical imbalance" in the brain being etiologic in pathologic behaviors. There are three general classes of neurotransmitters: biogenic amines, amino acids and peptides.

a. Biogenic Amines

(1) **Dopamine:**

(a) Major functions appear to be: experience of pleasure; and, to organize thoughts and feelings. Has a very significant role in the mediation of reward.

(b) Schizophrenia: associated with dopamine **hyperactivity.** The D_2 receptor is specifically implicated. New data on a D_3 receptor has potential implications for schizophrenia. The new antipsychotic medication, Clozapine, works at the D_4 receptor.

(c) Manic states: associated with dopamine **hyperactivity.**

(d) Depressed states: associated with dopamine **hypoactivity.**

(2)   **Norepinephrine:**

 (a) Major functions appears to be relative activation;

 (b) central role in **sleep** cycles and arousal;

 (c) involved with **anxiety and pain**;

 (d) also appears to be important in **anxiety** disorders.

 (e) MHPG (metabolite of norepinephrine) is lowered in urine of persons with severe **depressive** disorders.

 (f) MHPG in CSF is decreased in some persons who have attempted **suicide**.

(3)   **Serotonin:**

 (a) Major general functions associated with regulation of mood, sleep, pain, perception, aggression, memory, appetite, blood pressure, heart rate and respiration.

 (b) Dorsal raphe nucleus contains almost all of the brain's serotonergic cell bodies.

 (c) Some correlates with **schizophrenic** states.

 (d) **Depressed** states: associated with lowered serotonin levels.

 (e) 5-HIAA (metabolite of serotonin): low levels associated with **suicide** attempts in depressed persons.

 (f) 5-HIAA concentrations also lowered in persons who demonstrate **aggressive and violent** behaviors.

 (g) Associated with **anxiety**, including the **obsessive-compulsive** disorders.

 (h) Lowered levels associated with **sleep reduction**.

(4)   **Histamine**

 (a) Histamine cells are present in the hypothalamus.

      (b)   Major association is with the sleep-wake cycle.

      (c)   Abnormalities in the histaminic system have been observed in schizophrenic patients.

  (5)   **Acetylcholine**

      (a)   Major functions appears to be associated with sleep, aggression, <u>memory and cognition</u>.

      (b)   Implicated in mood disorders. Overactivity of cholinergic pathways associated with depression.

      (c)   Correlations with sleep problems.

      (d)   Degeneration of cholinergic neurons (nucleus basalis of Meynert) is observed in Alzheimer's disease, Down's syndrome and Parkinson's disease.

      (e)   Blockade of cholinergic receptors can result in delirium.

b. <u>Amino Acids</u>

  (1)   Gamma-aminobutyric acid (GABA)

      (a)   Major activity is mediating presynaptic inhibition through modulation of the chloride ions. Leads to calming effect.

      (b)   Account for 60% of synapses in the human brain.

      (c)   Decreased GABA activity is associated with development of **anxiety** and some forms of **epilepsy**.

      (d)   Correlations with **Tardive Dyskinesia**.

      (e)   Suggestions that underactivity may be correlated with the **schizophrenias**.

c. <u>Peptides</u>

  (1)   Major correlate is with the control of stress and pain.

  (2)   Some correlates with mood disorders (particularly Somatostatin; Substance P and Vasopressin).

       (3)   Enkephalins and endorphins have been correlated with schizophrenia.

       (4)   Some correlations with alcoholism.

3. **Genetics and Behavioral Variants**

   a. Much research has been done on inheritability of behaviors.

   b. The following behavioral conditions have some suggestion of genetic involvement.

      (1)   Schizophrenia
      (2)   Mood Disorders: Bipolar and Major Depressive Disorder
      (3)   Antisocial and Borderline Personality Disorders
      (4)   Alzheimer's Disease; Huntington's Chorea; Tourette's Syndrome
      (5)   Alcoholism and some other forms of chemical dependence
      (6)   Obsessive Compulsive Disorder; and, some other Anxiety Disorders (e.g., Panic Disorder)
      (7)   Enuresis and some Learning Disabilities
      (8)   Homosexuality

E. <u>Psychodynamic Considerations</u>

1. **"Freudian"**: the childhood experience of life is the paradigm for much that comes later. The following are basic concepts that are in common use today.

   a. <u>Pleasure principle</u>: people seek pleasure and avoid pain.

   b. <u>Libido</u>: "Psychic energy." This word has been misinterpreted to be sexual energy. While psychic energy can take a sexual form, libido is more than sexual.

   c. Pathologic problems arise from early "trauma".

      (1)   <u>Regression</u>: Under stress the person returns to an earlier maturational level at which the trauma occurred. E.g., if the child was traumatized in the Phallic stage, with stress (e.g., tired, ill, birth of another sibling), the child may give up the Phallic stage of adaptation and regress to an Anal stage and begin soiling again.

(2) <u>Fixation</u>: Due to trauma at a given stage of psychosexual development the person does not mature further in a psychological sense. Also fixation may be due to a close, paralyzing attachment to another person, such as mother or father.

d. <u>Levels of awareness</u>

(1) **Unconscious**: Material is out of the person's awareness; therefore, the person doesn't know what it is.

(2) **Preconscious**: the person is not presently aware of it, but with focus on the topic, can become aware. E.g., your telephone number is not in your awareness; however, with attention or concentration you can become aware of it.

(3) **Conscious Awareness**: the material of which the person is aware at the present time.

e. <u>Psychodynamic Mental Structures</u>

(1) **Id**: basically the instinctual drive, e.g., food, sex, etc.

(2) **Superego**: standards a person has, values. Is the conscience.

(3) **Ego**: many functions are in the ego. Mediates between Id and Superego.

   (a) Ego Functions: remember the mnemonic **ROADSIT**

     a) <u>R</u>eality Testing: ability to separate fact from fantasy.
     b) <u>O</u>bject Relations: ability to establish healthy interpersonal relations.
     c) <u>A</u>utonomous Functions: memory, perception, movement, IQ, singing, etc.
     d) <u>D</u>efenses: (covered in Section Three)
     e) <u>S</u>ynthesis: ability to integrate components into a statement of "This is who I am."
     f) <u>I</u>mpulse Control: delay of gratification.
     g) <u>T</u>hinking: Thought process and content.

The stronger the ego, the stronger the person.

(b) **Ego boundaries and "pathology":** Ego boundary is a concept which represents the separation of the host from the environment. If the ego boundaries are too rigid, an appropriate interchange with the environment is not possible (e.g., rigid rules against enjoying oneself). If they are too weak the environment may overwhelm the person; or, the person's internal impulses may be unleashed on the environment in an unmodulated form (e.g., primitive rage).

f. Transference: all aspects of the patient's feelings and behavior toward the therapist/doctor which are not elicited by the professional's behavior.

g. Counter-Transference: the emotional response of the therapist or doctor to the patient.

2. **Erikson's Psychodynamic Theory of Psychosocial Tasks**

a. Focuses on the individual's interchange with the environment/society. From this psychological--social interchange at certain ages and stages, and the conflict generated by this interchange, certain outcomes are predictable for the person.

b. The conflicts are described as bipolar (e.g. trust versus mistrust); however, this bipolar description represents the ends of a continuum. I.e., there are relative positions along the continuum at which the person may be placed dependent upon how well (relatively speaking) the conflict has been resolved.

c. In Erikson's theory there are eight tasks which a person must complete in a lifetime to have a totally full, normal life (See Table 1).

d. Problems can arise from an inadequate resolution of conflict at a given stage; and/or, later stages built on a poor foundation.

Table 1

Erikson's Eight Stages of Psychosocial Development

Stage	Age	Task	Comments
1.	0-18 mos.	Trust vs. Mistrust	Needs handled? Contiguity of own actions established?

"Basically it's safe"

2.	18 mos.- 3 yrs.	Autonomy vs. Shame and Doubt	Once he ventures out, what are his reactions and those of family; can he build a sense of standing on two feet without shame and doubt?

"I am an independent person and can determine some things"

3.	4-6 yrs.	Initiative vs. Guilt	Superego anger: overwhelming fear? Oedipus Complex constructively resolved?

"I can plan and others will not overwhelm all my planning"

4.	6-13 yrs.	Industry vs. Inferiority	School entrance; peer relationships; danger; sense of adequacy especially away from home and with equals.

"I have something to offer"

5.	11-20 yrs.	Sense of Identity vs. Role Confusion	Rapid changes, ambiguous period; task: maintain identity and incorporate changes.

"I know me and I can make it as an adult"

6.	20-35 yrs.	Intimacy vs. Isolation	Knows who he is; now must develop affiliation with others; intimacy with them.

"I can share my life and gain support from others"

7.	35-65 yrs.	Generativity vs. Stagnation	Guiding next generation, acquiring personal meaning in life, and making contribution.

"I have meaning and mean something to others"

8.	65-+ yrs.	Integrity vs. Despair	Maintain dignity of personal life.

"I am proud of my life"

F. Learning Theory

1. Major focus is on defective informational systems, poor training in life coping skills, poor training in the "facts of life" necessary for full functioning and adaptation in the social world.

2. **Learned Cognitive Distortions**

   a. Automatic negative thoughts, e.g., "Dummy", which have an attendant negative emotion accompanying the thought.

   b. Misperception of the world: "All men only want one thing.

3. **Learned attachment** of a given feeling to a situation. E.g., learned feared of elevators after once having been stuck on one in a burning building.

4. **Social Learning Theories**

   a. Focuses on learning through modeling after significant role models.

   b. Modeling in child abuse: most abusing adults were themselves abused as children. They are doing to children what they learned from their parents was "OK".

   c. Inner city gang behavior: peer pressure and role modeling by the significant others in the environment.

IV. **MILESTONES AND SIGNIFICANT PERSONS**

A. Pinel: Person who literally took the chains off the mentally ill in "insane asylums" in France; and demonstrated they were not dangerous persons who needed to be locked up.

B. Freud: Pioneered the issue that early (traumatic) experiences influenced the later life and development of pathologic behavior. Also documented the issue that there is a natural unfolding of human psychosexual developmental stages.

C. Erikson: Extended natural psychosocial developmental stages into the full spectrum of life from birth to death.

D. Beers: A lay person who had experienced a mental disorder. His hospitalization for that condition led him to champion outpatient care and the mental hygiene-mental health movement.

E. Freeman and Watts: Introduced prefrontal lobotomy in the USA. Post-surgery, patients reported a decrease in tension and psychotic-like symptoms.

F. Cerletti: Introduced Electro Convulsive Treatment (ECT) after the observation that some mentally ill epileptic patients had a clearing of their mental illness in the postictal state. This led to the hypothesis that if one gave the mentally ill person a seizure their mental illness might be relieved.

G. Modern Psychopharmacology: In 1949 & 1950 modern psychopharmacology was introduced and subsequently has appreciated a massive popularity and success in the amelioration of the more severe mental disorders.

V. PREVALENCE OF MENTAL DISORDERS

A. Household survey in Baltimore, New Haven and St. Louis (1988). Robbin, L., Myers, J., Shapiro, S. NIMH sponsored. A lifetime prevalence study. Major findings were:

1. Experienced alcohol abuse or dependence   13.6%

2. Other drug abuse and dependence   5.6%

3. Experienced phobias   11.3%

4. Experienced major depression   5.7%

B. Lifetime prevalence rates from five Epidemiologic Catchment Areas of the country. Regier and Associates.

1. Alcohol   13.3%

2. Drug abuse   5.9%

3. Anxiety disorders 14.6%

    a. Phobia   12.5%
    b. Panic   1.6%
    c. Obsess/comp   2.5%

    4. Major Depression   5.8%

    5. Dysthymia   3.3%

C. <u>Summary of findings from different sources</u>

    1. #1 mental disorder: alcohol abuse/dependency.

    2. If you combine all the anxiety disorders, they are the single #1 problem.

    3. #3 problem: <u>depression</u>. 5.7% experienced **major** depression.

    4. The three <u>LEAST</u> common disorders were:

        (1)   Schizophreniform
        (2)   Somatization
        (3)   Anorexia Nervosa

D. <u>Midtown Manhattan project (1954)</u> by Rennie and Srole.

    1. About 25% are seriously crippled by mental or emotional illness.

    2. About 55% additionally are mildly to moderately crippled but are able to function.

    3. Lower socio-economic-status (SES) people have six times the symptoms that other SES groups have. SES was seen to be the single most significant variable.

E. Suicide is the second leading cause of death among young persons aged 15-24. For black youth, homicide is the leading cause of death.

F. Men have higher rates of psychiatric disorders than women and a higher incidence of alcoholism and antisocial personality.

G. Major depression and phobias are more common among women.

H. The 25-44 age group has the highest rate of psychiatric disorders.

I. There is no difference in rates of disorders between blacks and whites.

J. Currently there are more patients occupying beds in <u>public</u> mental institutions than all other hospital beds combined. And, for every admission to a state hospital there is an admission to a private hospital.

K. At least one out of every ten individuals will spend some portion of his life in a psychiatric hospital.

L. One out of every four individuals will suffer an emotional or mental illness of such magnitude that medical treatment will be required. Does not include those with psychosomatic problems or those responding psychologically to physical illness.

M. The trend for the last few decades is a decrease in the number of persons who occupy hospital beds for emotional illness.

   NOTE: Admission rate has not changed--the length of stay has. This is secondary to appropriate medications being developed, managed health care, changes in third party payor reimbursements, and other community options being present.

N. <u>Socio-economic Status (SES) and Mental Illness</u>

   1. There is a high positive correlation between SES and Bipolar Disease as well as "neuroses."

   2. Psychosis is more prevalent in the lower SES.

   3. From the inner city to the suburbs, there is a positive correlation with mental HEALTH (<u>Hollingshead and Redlich, New Haven Study, 1952</u>).

O. In regard to the overall treatment of the mentally ill:

   60% cared for by primary care physicians.
   20% cared for by trained mental health professional.
   20% get no treatment at all.

CHAPTER 2

DIAGNOSIS AND INTERVENTION

I. **GENERAL CONSIDERATIONS**

A. Until recently the field of Psychiatry has had to rely upon trained and quantified observations of "behavior" to establish diagnoses.

B. Because behavior is pathoplastic, and the same behavior can emanate from a wide variety of different sources, a complete physical examination with laboratory tests of total functioning of the person is mandatory for an adequate workup.

C. With the advent of neuro-imaging techniques a more refined diagnostic procedure has been introduced to the field of Psychiatry. The limits of the utility of neuro-imaging have yet to be established.

II. **INTERVIEWING AS A DIAGNOSTIC TOOL**

A. <u>General stance in interviewing</u>: non-critical, non-leading, data gathering.

B. <u>Interview styles</u>

1. Associative

a. Interviewer says (verbally and non-verbally) the least in order to allow the patient to get on with their agenda. Generally, the best way to open an interview is a nod, or "What brings you to see me?"

b. Interviewer associates their next question to what the patient brings up. Generally leads to highest compliance rate from patients in their treatment.

c. It is often said that in the first two minutes of an associative interview the patient will present the central core of the issues involved.

2. Laundry list

a. Interviewer structures interview with preset questions to get specific data. Rarely helpful in dealing with the practice of Psychiatry.

b. Misses a great deal of the patient's agenda and gives the impression of "I know what's important, you don't".

C. <u>Concepts in interviewing</u>

1.   **Support:**   A response that shows interest in, concern for, or understanding of the patient.

2.   **Reassurance:**   A response that tends to establish the sense of merit, well-being, or self-reliance in the patient.

3.   **Empathy:**   A response that recognizes or names the patient's feeling and does not criticize it.   Accepts patient's feeling even though interviewer may believe the feeling to be wrong.

4.   **Confrontation:**   A response by the interviewer that points out to the patient his feeling, behavior, or previous statement.

5.   **Reflection:**   A response that repeats, mirrors, or echoes a portion of what the patient just said.

6.   **Interpretation:**   A confrontation that is based upon an inference rather than upon an observation.

7.   **Silence:**   A communication, a response. A silent response can show interest, withdrawal, lack of interest, support, or it can show that the doctor is not listening.   Most useful are the supportive silence and the interested silence.

8.   **Summation:**   A response that reviews patient's information

D. The interviewer can make the patient defensive by:

1. Not listening
2. Judging (critical parent)
3. Being a "Know-it-all"
4. Assuming or implying something is true
5. Lecturing
6. Talking <u>to</u> or <u>at</u>, not <u>with</u>

E. The interviewer can assist the flow of the interview by:

1. Asking the least leading question possible
2. Focusing on the feelings
3. Clarifying patients' communications
4. Get congruence on what the patient is thinking and feeling.

III. MENTAL STATUS EXAMINATION

Sometimes described as the "physical examination of the mind." It is a way of organizing and documenting observations. An outline of the "functional mind" at the time of the interview. Components are as follows:

A. Appearance and Behavior

1. General Description of the person as they are encountered in the interview.

2. Psychomotor Activity: Posture and speech. Includes eye contact.

3. Expressive Mannerisms: unique and repeated words or gestures that are distinctive to that person.

4. Attitude: Cooperativeness; Contact and Rapport (can you understand the world of the person and can you establish emotional contact with them?).

B. Sensorium: Dysfunction here suggests an organic condition.

1. Consciousness: Level and fluctuations

2. Orientation: Person, Place, Time and Situation

3. Memory:

    a. Immediate: recall three unrelated things in the interview.

    b. Recent: Current news events (2 weeks)

    c. Remote: Old, verifiable data (e.g. What date was Pearl Harbor bombed? In what city was President Kennedy shot?)

4. Attention and concentration: Can they attend to the interview; and, can they logically problem solve (Serial 7's).

C. Thought process

1. Production of thought: pressured, blocked, retarded, fragmented.

2. Continuity of thought: looseness of associations, tangential, circumstantial, clang associations, word salad, etc..

D. <u>Thought Content and Intellect</u>

    1. Relationship to reality: autistic, delusional, etc..

       a. Sense of reality

       b. Reality Testing

       c. Adaptation to reality

    2. Concept formation: abstract or concrete--can the person interpret proverbs, or does the individual simply reword the proverb.

    3. Topics and Issues: what is the content focus of the patient's verbal productions; e.g. "someone is trying to harm me."

    4. Morbid preoccupations: phobias; obsessions; suicidal thought, feelings or impulses; homicidal thoughts feelings or impulses.

    5. Values and Ideals: What are the standards by which the person lives their life. What kind of person does the individual want to be? How should children be raised?

    6. General Intellect: estimated from general fund of information, vocabulary. Below average, average, or above average.

    7. Insight and Judgment: do they understand the cause of illness; social judgement.

E. <u>Perceptual disturbances</u>

    1. Hallucinations

    2. Illusions

F. <u>Emotional Regulation</u>

    1. Subjective evidence for emotions: what patient reports

    2. Objective evidence for emotions: what the interviewer observes.

    3. Appropriateness of the emotions: does the emotion fit the topic?

4. Ambivalence: two opposing feelings towards significant others at the same time.

5. Depersonalization/derealization: _feeling_ that there is something "amiss" with the self or the world.

G. Volition:

1. Energy/spontaneity

2. Will

3. Goal directedness

H. Somatic Functioning:

1. Sleep changes.

2. Appetite changes.

3. Weight changes which are unplanned.

4. Changes in libido or interest in pleasurable activities.

5. As noted above, a physical examination should be a part of a total work up of a given patient.

IV. **DIAGNOSTIC AND STATISTICAL MANUAL OF MENTAL DISORDERS: THIRD EDITION, REVISED (DSM-III-R).**

A. The Diagnostic and Statistical Manual:

1. Atheoretical and with few exceptions (e.g., substance abuse disorders) does not imply etiology.

2. Codification of disorders by **groups of symptoms.** Specific inclusion and exclusion criteria must be satisfied before a DSM-III-R diagnosis is made.

B. Multiaxial system

1. **Axis I:** All mental disorders except personality disorders

2. **Axis II:** Personality Disorders; and specific childhood developmental disorders.

3. **Axis III:** Physical disorders and conditions

4. **Axis IV:** Severity of symptomatology

5. **Axis V:** Highest level of adaptive functioning in the last year.

AXES IV & V are basically research tools.

V. **LABORATORY DATA**

A. General Tests

1. Complete Blood Count (CBC); Hematocrit and Hemoglobin

2. Thyroid Function: thyroid dysfunction can produce profound emotional effects.

3. Blood sugar: hypo- and hyper-glycemic conditions can present with depressive, aggressive and anxiety symptoms.

4. Electrolytes: imbalance can have massive emotional effects.

5. Blood urea nitrogen (BUN): renal studies are particularly important for persons to be placed on psychotropic medications.

6. Liver Function: disrupted in many mental conditions particularly those that are Organic Mental Disorders; Substance Abuse Disorders; and as a consequence of certain psychotropic medication use.

B. Special tests

1. Screening tests for sexually transmitted diseases. Neurosyphilis and infections such as Human Immuno Deficiency Virus have dementing possibilities.

2. Urine screening tests for drugs of abuse. Toxicity on many recreational drugs can present a picture that is similar to a wide variety of mental disorders.

VI. BRAIN IMAGING

A. <u>Structural brain imaging</u>: beginning to replace older more invasive and uncomfortable procedures like pneumoencephalograms. Exams static brain structure.

1. **Computer Tomography (CT)**

   a. Data from X-ray of brain stored in computer.

   b. Computer manipulation of the data stored can then visually reconstruct the brain. Computer can be asked to reproduce given sections of the brain.

   c. Utility: for examining bone and calcified regions of the brain; and examining for ventricular enlargement.

   d. Disadvantage: can't tell grey versus white matter. Some areas of brain are difficult to image with CT. Can only image in transverse planes.

   e. Abnormalities are often observed in Schizophrenia, Anorexia Nervosa, Alcoholism, and Dementia. Results are equivocal with mood disorders.

2. **Magnetic Resonance Imaging, (MRI)**

   a. A strong magnetic field is applied to the brain.

   b. Characteristic electromagnetic energy patterns are released.

   c. Energy patterns are computer analyzed to give a visual image of the brain.

   d. Utility: can differentiate grey versus white matter.

   e. Disadvantage: can't distinguish bony structures or calcifications. Can't be used with persons who have significant metal objects in their body, e.g., skull plate.

   f. Abnormalities have been documented in Schizophrenia, Childhood Autism, and some equivocal data in Bipolar Disorder.

B. <u>Functional neuro-imaging</u>: Yields information regarding how regional areas of the brain are <u>performing</u> from a metabolic standpoint. Operates on the premise that brain regions that are more active have more blood flow.

1. **Positron Emission Tomography, (PET)**

   a. Compounds labeled with positron emitting isotopes are injected into the person.

   b. In the brain, the emitted positrons interact with electrons and emit gamma rays that are picked up by the PET camera and stored in computers.

   c. Can be used to study the characteristics (including density) of neurotransmitter receptors in the brain; and, to study glucose and oxygen metabolization.

   d. Demonstrated changes have been documented in Schizophrenia, Alzheimer's Disease, Obsessive-Compulsive Disorder, Bipolar Disorder, seizures, and stroke.

   e. Very expensive.

2. **Single Photon Emission Computer Tomography, (SPECT)**

   a. Uses single photon emitting isotopes with longer half-life than those used in PET.

   b. Due to longer half-life can study brain function for longer periods of time.

   c. Resolution isn't as good as with PET.

   d. Mainly used for regional blood flow studies at this time.

   e. Very useful in stroke characterization. Some application in Alzheimer's Disease diagnosis; and, the establishment of other dementing disorders.

   f. Less expensive than PET.

VII. PSYCHOLOGICAL AND NEUROPSYCHOLOGICAL ASSESSMENT

A. <u>Intelligence Tests</u> - These are the most structured of all psychological tests.

1. The most popular and the most valid for adults is the Wechsler Adult Intelligence Scale-Revised (WAIS-R); for young children, the <u>Stanford-Binet</u> is most valid; and for older children and adolescents, the Wechsler Intelligence Scale for Children-Revised (WISC-R) is the most valid. IQ scores are generally distributed in the following manner.

   a. Less than or equal to 69 = mentally defective
   b. 70 to 79 = borderline intelligence
   c. 80 to 89 = dull normal
   d. 90 to 109 = average
   e. 110 to 119 = bright normal
   f. 120 to 129 = superior
   g. Greater than or equal to 130 = very superior or genius.

   NOTE: IQ test scores are highly correlated with education.

B. <u>Achievement tests</u>: Achievement tests have been developed to assess the amount of material which an individual has accomplished. E.g., with children there are tests that examine reading, spelling, and arithmetic skills of the child, and compare the child's scores to National norms. The most popular for the general public is the <u>Wide Range Achievement Test</u> (WRAT)

C. <u>Neuropsychological Tests</u>: These are used to evaluate the integrity of the brain.

1. **The Halstead-Reitan Neuropsychological Test Battery is the most complete, reliable and valid psychological assessment of brain functioning.**

   a. In the hands of a well trained Neuropsychologist the battery of tests can provide a very accurate assessment of the functioning of the brain. It can yield statements of selective deficits associated with specific areas of the brain; and, can make statements regarding the brain's functioning as a whole.

   b. This battery is often used as a non-invasive mechanism to track the recovery of neuropsychological function after brain insult.

    c. It is particularly useful in establishing dysfunction in conditions which, at the present time, do not readily lend themselves to biological assessment (e.g., Alzheimer's Disease).

    d. This battery of tests is very useful in the differential diagnostic question of whether a given symptom complex is on the basis of organic or functional etiology.

2. **The Luria**

    a. Assesses: memory; rhythm; tactile, auditory and visual functioning; receptive and expressive speech; writing, spelling, reading, and arithmetic.

    b. Focuses on the identification of types of cognitive problems with little emphasis on locus of brain dysfunction.

3. **The Bender Gestalt**

    a. Tests for visual-motor coordination.

    b. Can reflect gross brain dysfunction so is useful as a screening tool; but, has limited value as a differential diagnostic instrument for specific brain location dysfunction.

D. <u>Personality/Pathology Testing</u>

1. Tests which assess dimensions of an individual's personality. They are typically divided into <u>subjective</u> versus <u>objective</u> personality tests.

    a. <u>Subjective</u> personality tests (Projective tests): have been developed from theories, e.g. psychoanalytic theory, and typically assume the "projective hypothesis." The <u>projective hypothesis</u>: when a person is faced with an ambiguous situation, they will project their own internal structure onto the external ambiguous situation. Therefore, we assume if a person is given an ambiguous stimulus, they will project their internal structure onto the ambiguous stimulus.

    The major subjective personality tests are:

    (1) **Rorschach:** This test consists of ten (10) very ambiguous ink-blots which presumably taps the unconscious dimensions of a person's personality functioning.

(2) **Thematic Apperception Test (TAT):** Consists of more structured stimulus pictures which are vague in content. The person is asked to make up a story about the picture. The story presumably reveals information about preconscious personality.

Advantages of subjective-projective tests: They pick up idiosyncratic themes. They are more difficult to fake good or fake bad.

Disadvantages of subjective-projective tests: These require a well trained and skilled clinical psychologist for interpretation of the test results. They are labor intensive, difficult to score reliably, and subject to misinterpretation.

b. <u>Objective tests</u> are developed statistically without regard to theory. The most used of these is the Minnesota Multiphasic Personality Inventory (MMPI-2).

(1) The clinical scales on the MMPI-2 are: Hypochondriasis, Depression, Hysteria, Psychopathic Deviate, Masculinity-Femininity, Paranoia, Schizophrenia, Mania, Social Introversion.

(2) The MMPI provides information on symptom levels--not diagnosis. It also yields information about defensive structures and test taking defensiveness.

(3) The MMPI is **NOT** a test of personality; rather it is a test of pathology

2. **Self Rating Scales:** these are very subject to purposeful distortion by the person taking the test. There are a very large number of these. Probably the most widely used is:

a. <u>The Beck Depression Inventory (BDI)</u> takes about five minutes to administer and can be used in a wide variety of medical settings.

BDI scoring:

0-10	not depressed
11-20	mildly depressed
21-30	moderately depressed
31-40	severely depressed
> 40	depressed but exaggerating the extent of the depression

3. Objective tests and self rating scales generally are easier to administer and to score. They are less labor intensive. They generally have higher reliability.

   They are easier to fake good or fake bad.

E. Special Tests:

1. There are a series of psychological instruments constructed for very specific purposes.

   a. Freedman and Rosenman: A & B Behavior Patterns

      A Type = "running out of time"; correlated with coronary heart disease

   b. The State-Trait Anxiety Scale: measures how much anxiety a person has as a specific response to a given state or situation; versus how much anxiety is a part of the persons general personality (trait).

VIII. FLOW CHART OF DIFFERENTIAL DIAGNOSIS

```
                        "Abnormal Behavior"
                                |
            ┌───────────────────┴───────────────────┐
        Psychotic                               Nonpsychotic
            |                                        |
     ┌──────┴──────┐                         ┌───────┴───────┐
  Organic      Nonorganic                 Organic       Nonorganic
     |             |                          |              |
   ┌─Acute      ┌─Thought Disorder         ┌─Acute          |
   └─Chronic    |                          └─Chronic         |
               |                                             |
               |                                          ┌─Bother Others
               ├─Brief Reactive                           |  └─Personality
               |  Psychosis                               |     Disorders
               |                                          |
               ├─Schizophreniform                         |
               |                                          |
               ├─Schizophrenia                            └─Bother Self
               |                                             |
               ├─Schizo-affective                           ├─"Neuroses"
               |                                             |   Anxiety Disorders
               ├─Delusional                                 |   Dissociative Disordr.
               |  Disorder                                  |   Somatoform Disordr.
               |                                             |
               ├─Induced Psychiatric                        ├─Psychological
               |  Disorder                                  |   Factors Affecting
               |                                             |   Physical Conditions
               └─Not otherwise specified                    |
               |                                             ├─Adjustment Disorders
             └─Affective Disorder                            |
               |                                             └─Minor Affective
               ├─Bipolar Disorder                                Disorders
               |
               └─Major Affective
                  Disorder
```

CHAPTER 3

MANAGEMENT OF MENTAL DISORDERS

WE ARE PLACING INFORMATION ABOUT PATIENT MANAGEMENT AT THIS POINT
SO THE STUDENT HAS THE INFORMATION TO APPLY TOWARDS CARE OF
INDIVIDUALS WITH DIFFERENT DISORDERS.

I. **COMPLIANCE** (also called adherence):

A. Approximately 30-35% of patients fail to comply either in
part or completely.

B. Persons who don't comply well.

1. Chronic illness: Big 3 are Cardiovascular, Mental
Disorders and Arthritis/rheumatoid
2. Long term maintenance
3. Preventive medications for conditions that have no overt
symptoms (e.g., hypertension).
4. If D/C, only gives subtle or remote effects
5. Children, elderly, and disadvantaged
6. Hostile
7. Risk takers
8. Hypochondriacs

C. Good M.D.-Patient relation produces good compliance.
M.D.'s who get good compliance:

1. Talks with patient about how patient feels about
treatment.
2. M.D.'s attitudes toward drugs as well as patient
3. Gives close supervision
4. Patient likes the doctor and satisfied with management.

D. Poor relation produces: M.D. shopping, going to non-M.D.,
increased malpractice actions, increases in depression in
the patients.

E. Variables affecting if a treatment regimen is followed.

1. Easy to learn
2. Easy to carry out
3. Takes little time
4. Doesn't lead to social isolation
5. Decrease fear in the patient
6. Patient believes is ill

F. Medications compliance

1. Correlate with daily activities, e.g. meals
2. As few as possible; less than or equal to 3 times/day

3. As infrequent as possible; less than or equal to 4 times/day
4. Few side effects
5. NOT PRN
6. Meaning of medications to the patient: e.g. more drugs = sick

II. **PSYCHOPHARMACOLOGY**

A. General Comments.

1. The goal of therapy is usually reduction of symptoms. Frequently, psychopharmacological agents are used adjunctively.

2. **Psychopharmacology has dramatically decreased the length of hospitalization for the major psychiatric disorders. It has decreased the degree of suffering from both psychotic and non-psychotic disorders.**

3. **There are four major classes of psychotropics: Antipsychotics; Anti-depressants; Anti-manics/Mood Stabilizers; and the Anxiolytics/Sedative-Hypnotics.**

B. Antipsychotic Drugs: (neuroleptics; "major tranquilizers")

1. **Classes**

   a. Phenothiazines: tricyclic structure with different side chains

      (1)   aliphatic: chlorpromazine (Thorazine)

      (2)   piperidine: thioridazine (mellaril), mesoridazine (Serentil).

      (3)   piperazine: trifluoperazine (Stelazine), fluphenazine (Prolixin), perphenazine (Trilafon).

   b. Butyrophenones

      (1)   Haloperidol (Haldol)

   c. Thioxanthenes

      (1)   Thiothixene (Navane)

   d. Dihydroindolones

      (1)   Molindone (Moban)

   e. <u>Dibenzoxazepines</u>

      (1)   Loxapine (Loxitane)

   f. <u>Diphenylbutylpiperidines</u>

      (1)   Pimozide (Orap)

   g. <u>Dibenzodiazepines</u>

      (1)   Clozapine (Clozaril)

2. **Indications for Use**

   a. <u>Schizophrenia</u>

      (1)   Acute - control of psychotic symptoms

      (2)   Chronic - maintenance; relapse prevention

   b. <u>Brief Reactive Psychosis</u>

      (1)   Acute

   c. <u>Delusional Disorder</u>

   d. <u>Mania</u>

      (1)   Acute - adjunctive with lithium until psychotic symptoms remit and lithium levels reach therapeutic range

   e. <u>Major Depression with Psychotic Features</u>

      (1)   Acute - adjunctive with antipsychotics until psychotic symptoms remit

   f. <u>Organic Mental Syndromes</u>

      (1)   Delirium

      (2)   Dementia

   g. <u>Borderline Personality Disorder</u> - especially rage and recurrent "micro-psychotic" episodes

   h. <u>Tourette's Syndrome</u>

   i. <u>Huntington's Disease</u>

   j. <u>Behavior Problems with Mental Retardation</u>

3. **Mode of Action**

   a. <u>Blockade of post-synaptic dopamine (mostly D_2) receptors</u>. (Clozapine preferentially blocks D_4 receptors).

   b. Degree of blockade directly correlated to clinical potency (high to low).

   c. Low potency drugs more often associated with sedative, anticholinergic, and orthostatic hypotensive side effects.

   d. <u>Major dopamine pathways involved</u>.

      (1)   Mesolimbic/mesocortical (limbic system, cortex)

      (2)   Nigrostriatal (basal ganglion)

      (3)   Tuberoinfundibular (pituitary)

   e. <u>Also block other post-synaptic receptors</u>.

      (1)   Norepinephrine (NE)

      (2)   Acetylcholine (Ach)

      (3)   Histamine (H)

4. **Side Effects**

   a. <u>Sedation</u>

      (1)   Due to histamine (H_1) blockade.

      (2)   More common with aliphatic and piperidine phenothiazines and other low potency, high dosage drugs.

      (3)   Tolerance can be achieved

      (4)   Give one dose at bedtime if possible

   b. <u>Anticholinergic</u>

      (1)   Due to cholinergic receptor blockade (muscarinic)

      (2)   More common in aliphatic and piperidine phenothiazines.

      (3)   Tolerance can be achieved.

    (4)   More problems in the elderly.

    (5)   Examples

        (a)   Dry Mouth

        (b)   Constipation

        (c)   Urinary hesitancy and retention

        (d)   Blurred vision (near vision)

        (e)   Exacerbation of glaucoma

    (6)   Treat with neostigmine or bethanechol.

c. <u>Orthostatic Hypotension</u>

    (1)   Due to $alpha_1$-adrenergic blockade

    (2)   More common in aliphatic and piperidine phenothiazines.

    (3)   Important in treating elderly patients.

    (4)   Use norepinephrine (Levophed) or a pure alpha-adrenergic stimulator.

    (5)   <u>Do not use epinephrine</u>: is a beta-adrenergic stimulant and can make hypotension worse.

d. <u>Acute dystonia</u>

    (1)   An early extrapyramidal symptom (EPS).

    (2)   Occurs within the first 2-5 days of treatment.

    (3)   Involuntary sustained muscle contraction

    (4)   Usually involves jaw muscles, neck (torticollis), tongue, truck (opisthotonos), extraocular muscles (oculogyric crisis), dysphagia.

    (5)   Young males most susceptible

    (6)   Due to basal ganglia D_2 receptor blockade

    (7)   Treat with IM or IV antiparkinson agents.

    (8)   More common with high potency drugs.

e. <u>Parkinsonism</u> (Pseudoparkinson)

    (1)   Usually occurs within the first 1-4 weeks of treatment.

    (2)   Bradykinesia or akinesia, shuffling gate, rigidity, masked facies, tremor.

    (3)   Treat with oral antiparkinson agents and/or lowering dosage of antipsychotic.

    (4)   More common with high-potency drugs

    (5)   Due to basal ganglia D_2 receptor blockade

    (6)   More common in older patients

f. <u>Akathisia</u>

    (1)   Motor restlessness, dysphoria, fidgeting

    (2)   Due to basal ganglia D_2 receptor blockade.

    (3)   Usually occurs between 1-8 weeks of treatment

    (4)   Often confused with anxiety or psychotic agitation.

    (5)   Doesn't respond will to antiparkinson drugs

    (6)   Treat with beta-blockers (Inderal) or benzodiazepines (Ativan).

    (7)   More common with high potency drugs.

g. <u>"Rabbit Syndrome"</u>

    (1)   Perioral tremor

    (2)   Rare, late appearing

    (3)   May respond to antiparkinson drugs.

h. <u>Tardive Dyskinesia</u>: **VERY IMPORTANT**

    (1)   Late appearing

    (2)   Involuntary, slow choreiform or tic-like movements of the tongue, lips, facial muscles, limbs and trunk.

     (3)   Often presents with tongue protrusion, lip smacking, grimacing, chewing, eye-blinking.

     (4)   Usually develops after long-term, moderate to high dosage antipsychotic use.

     (5)   Presents as a break-through symptom or after dosage reduction.

     (6)   Probably due to denervation hypersensitivity of post-synaptic D_2 receptors.

     (7)   Risk increased in elderly, pre-existing brain damage, females, affective disorders.

     (8)   **May be permanent even with drug discontinuation**.

     (9)   Doesn't respond to antiparkinson drugs.

     (10)   May be helped with benzodiazepines, reserpine and dosage reduction of antipsychotic.

     (11)   Regular assessment by Abnormal Involuntary Movement Scale (AIMS) helps with early detection and prevention.

     (12)   Informed consent for use of these medications is very important.

i. <u>Agranulocytosis and leukopenia</u>

     (1)   usually seen with aliphatic and piperidine phenothiazine and most importantly with <u>clozapine</u>.

     (2)   Rate of 1-3% with clozapine, rare with others.

     (3)   Usually occurs within the first 2-4 months of treatment.

     (4)   Idiosyncratic: not related to dosage.

     (5)   Elderly women at greatest risk

     (6)   Monitoring of WBC is very important.

     (7)   Can present as fever, sore throat, infections.

j. <u>Photosensitivity</u>

     (1)   Usually seen with Thorazine

(2) Not dose related

(3) Severe sunburn possible

(4) Use sunscreen and limit UV exposure

k. Weight Gain

(1) Occurs with increased appetite

(2) More common with low potency drugs

l. Endocrine Effects

(1) Amenorrhea

(2) Galactorrhea

(3) Gynecomastia

(4) Decreased libido

(5) Impotence and ejaculatory problems in men due to alpha$_1$-adrenergic blockade (Mellaril).

(6) Due to dopamine blockade in pituitary and consequent hyperprolactinemia.

(7) Most often seen with low potency drugs.

(8) May be treated with amantadine (Symmetrel).

m. Ocular Effects

(1) Retinitis pigmentosa with Mellaril at dosages greater than 800 mg/d

(2) Can lead to blindness

n. Dermatologic Effects

(1) Especially with Thorazine

(2) Blue-gray skin discoloration in areas exposed to the sun.

(3) Often long-term, high-dose treatment.

o. Neuroleptic Malignant Syndrome

(1) Potentially fatal if not treated

     (2)   Muscle rigidity ("lead pipe"), fever, autonomic dysfunction, confusion.

     (3)   Incidence 1%

     (4)   Mortality rate about 20%

     (5)   More common with high potency drugs.

     (6)   Use with lithium may increase the risk.

     (7)   Occurs early after beginning treatment or increasing dose.

     (8)   May also have increase WBC, CPK.

     (9)   Concurrent illness common

     (10)   Treat by immediately stopping antipsychotics, supportive care, and possibly specific drugs such as bromocriptine or dantrolene. Consider using ECT.

5. Use in the Elderly

a. <u>Increased sensitivity to side effects</u>

     (1)   Sedation-confusion

     (2)   Hypotension leading to falls

     (3)   Anticholinergic: confusion, urinary retention, constipation.

b. More problems with low potency than with high potency drugs.

6. Use in pregnancy

a. Avoid if possible

b. No known teratogenic effects.

c. Use high potency drugs if needed

d. Are secreted in breast milk.

7. Drug Interactions

a. Sedative effects are additive

b. Anticholinergic effects are additive

8. General Treatment Principles

   a. All antipsychotics are equally effective in equivalent dosages.

   b. Side effects and potency are important in choosing one drug over another.

   c. Patient and family history of response helpful.

   d. More effective on <u>positive</u> symptoms of psychosis; less effective on <u>negative</u> symptoms.

   e. Treatment resistant patients should be offered a trial of clozapine; 30-40% of patients benefit.

   f. Depot or long-acting injectable agents (Prolixin, Haldol) useful in non-compliant patients.

C. <u>Antidepressants</u>

1. **Classes**

   a. <u>Heterocyclic (tricyclic)</u>

     (1)   Tertiary amines

       (a)   amitriptyline (Elavil)

       (b)   imipramine (Tofranil)

       (c)   doxepin (Sinequan)

       (d)   clomipramine (Anafranil)

       (e)   trimipramine (Surmontil)

     (2)   Secondary amines

       (a)   desipramine (Norpramin) (norepinephrine re-uptake blockade)

       (b)   nortriptyline (Pamelor)

       (c)   protriptyline (Vivactil)

   b. <u>Heterocyclic (tetracyclic)</u>

     (1)   Amoxapine (Asendin)

     (2)   Maprotiline (Ludiomil)

c. <u>Atypical</u>

    (1)   Trazodone (Desyrel) (serotonin re-uptake blockade)

    (2)   Fluoxetine (Prozac) (serotonin re-uptake blockade)

    (3)   Sertroline (Zoloft) (serotonin re-uptake blockade)

    (4)   Bupropion (Wellbutrin) (dopamine re-uptake blockade)

d. <u>Monoamine Oxidase Inhibitors (MAOI)</u>

    (1)   Hydrazine

        (a)   Isocarboxazid (Marplan)

        (b)   Phenelzine (Nardil)

    (2)   Non-hydrazine

        (a)   Tranylcypromine (Parnate)

2. **Indications for Use**

a. <u>Major depression</u>

    (1)   Single episode or recurrent

    (2)   Especially with vegetative symptoms

b. <u>Bipolar disorder, depressed</u>

    (1)   For acute use

    (2)   Chronic use may lead to rapid cycling

c. <u>Dysthymia</u>

d. <u>Atypical depression</u>

    (1)   Especially MAOI, serotonergic drugs

e. <u>Panic disorder</u>

f. <u>Obsessive-Compulsive Disorder</u>

    (1)   Clomipramine or fluoxetine

g. <u>Phobic Disorders</u>

    (1)   Agoraphobia

    (2)   Social Phobia: global

    (3)   Especially MAOI, serotonergic drugs

h. <u>Enuresis</u>

i. <u>School refusal/separation anxiety</u>

j. <u>Attention Deficit Hyperactivity Disorder (ADHD)</u>

k. <u>Chronic Pain</u>

l. <u>Bulimia nervosa</u>

    (1)   Especially serotonin re-uptake inhibitors

m. <u>Behavioral dyscontrol in brain-injured and mentally retarded</u>

n. <u>Narcolepsy/cataplexy</u>

o. <u>Organic affective disorders</u>

3. **Mode of action**

a. <u>Heterocyclics and Atypical agents</u>

    (1)   Differs from one agent to another

    (2)   Increase levels of CNS NE, 5-HT, DA between neurons by blocking re-uptake into the presynaptic neuron; immediate effect.

    (3)   Beta-adrenergic receptors (post-synaptic) are decreased in number and sensitivity (down-regulated); chronic effect.

    (4)   5HT system must be intact for down regulation of beta-adrenergic receptors to occur.

    (5)   Time line of chronic receptor changes follows that of clinical therapeutic effect.

b. <u>MAOI</u>

    (1)   Irreversible inhibition of MAO: entire body (CNS, gut, blood, etc.)

(2)   MAO needed for oxidation of the biogenic amines DA, NE, 5-HT, tyramine.

(3)   Increase in CNS 5-HT and NE with MAO blockade.

(4)   Occurs intracellularly.

4. **Side effects-Heterocyclics and Atypical** (As a rule, tertiary agents have more side effects than secondary, and atypical agents have fewer and more idiosyncratic side-effects.)

a. <u>Anticholinergic</u>

(1)   Dry mouth

(2)   Constipation

(3)   Sweating

(4)   Blurred vision

(5)   Tachycardia

(6)   Urinary hesitancy\retention

(7)   Delirium (toxic)

(8)   Impotence

b. <u>Sedation</u>

(1)   Due to <u>histamine</u> (H_1), serotonin, and cholinergic blockade

c. <u>Weight gain</u>

(1)   Due to <u>histamine</u> (H_2) blockade

(2)   Craving for carbohydrates

d. <u>Cardiac</u> - most important in mortality and morbidity

(1)   Orthostatic hypotension - due to $alpha_1$ adrenergic blockade (nortriptyline has the least)

(2)   Tachycardia, palpitations

(3)   Conduction changes: quinidine-like action

(4)   Arrhythmias

e. <u>CNS</u>

    (1)   Restlessness

    (2)   Insomnia   Seen more often with atypical drugs and desipramine

    (3)   Agitation

    (4)   Tremor

    (5)   Mania

    (6)   Seizures (especially with maprotiline)

    (7)   EPS similar to antipsychotics (amoxapine, due to D_2 blockade)

f. <u>Others</u>

    (1)   Skin rash

    (2)   Worsening of glaucoma

    (3)   Priapism (especially Trazadone)

5. **Side effects - MAOI**

a. <u>Hypertensive episodes</u>

    (1)   Usually due to tyramine in food or sympathomimetic drugs

    (2)   Compliance essential

b. <u>Interactive with narcotics</u> (especially meperidine [Demerol])

    (1)   Fever, headache, hypertension, agitation, seizures, coma

c. <u>Orthostatic hypotension</u>

d. <u>Orgasmic inhibition</u>

e. <u>Paresthesias</u> - possibly due to B6 reduction

f. <u>Insomnia</u>

g. <u>Mania</u>

h. <u>Weight gain</u>

6. Use in the Elderly

a. "Start low and go slow"

b. Hypotension a major problem (falls with resulting fractures) as are anticholinergic side effects, sedation/confusion

7. Use in Pregnancy

a. Avoid use in first trimester if possible

b. All agents are secreted in breast milk

8. Drug Interactions

a. CNS depression synergistic

b. Anticholinergic side effects can be synergistic

c. Hypertension with sympathomimetic drugs

9. General Treatment Principles

a. All antidepressant drugs are equally effective

b. They differ in mode of action, side effects and toxicity

c. 60-70% of depressed patients improve

d. Past personal and/or family history of drug response may predict future drug response

e. Clinical significance of selective neurotransmitter effects not clear

f. Some depressive subtypes (atypical, SAD, etc.) may respond better to serotonergic agents or MAO inhibitors

g. Most important reasons for poor patient response are: incorrect diagnosis, too low a dosage, too short a trial, side effect intolerance

h. After acute episode remits, maintenance for around 9-12 months at lowest effective dosage

i. If treatment resistant, options include: changing drugs, augmenting with lithium or thyroid hormones, ECT

j. Fluoxetine and trazadone safer in overdose; most others dangerous in overdose

k. Phobic - anxiety patients may respond to lower doses than needed for depressed patients

l. Usually must combine antidepressant with anti-psychotic for resolution of psychotic depressive episode

m. Trazadone good at improving sleep quality; often used with serotonergic drugs which have side effect of insomnia

n. Blood levels important with nortriptyline (has a therapeutic window 50-150 mg/ml)

D. <u>Lithium/Mood stabilizers</u>

   1. **Classes**

      a. <u>Lithium Carbonate</u>

      b. <u>Anticonvulsants</u>

         (1)   Carbamazepine (Tegretol)

         (2)   Valproic acid (Depakote, Depakene)

         (3)   Clonazepam (Klonopin)

      c. <u>Calcium channel blockers</u>

         (1)   Verapamil (Calan, Isoptin) - most commonly used in psychiatry

         (2)   Diltiazem (Cardizem)

         (3)   Nifedipine (Procardia)

   2. **Indications for use**

      a. <u>Bipolar Disorder</u>

         (1)   Acute, manic

         (2)   Chronic, mania and depression

      b. <u>Schizo-affective disorder</u>

      c. <u>Adjunct with antidepressant in non-responders.</u>

    d. <u>Behavioral dyscontrol in mental retardation; rage disorders</u>

    e. <u>Bulimia nervosa</u>

    f. <u>PMS</u>

3. **Mode of action**

    a. <u>Lithium</u>

        (1) Blocks inositol-1-phosphatase inside neurons

        (2) This blockade reduces the formation of phosphatidylinositolbisphosphate

        (3) Results in decreased response to neuro-transmitters in second messenger system

    b. <u>Carbamazepine</u>

        (1) Probably through regulation of calcium channels

        (2) May also have an effect on kindling in some neurons of the limbic system

    c. <u>Anticonvulsants</u>

        (1) May potentiate GABA ergic neurotransmission

        (2) May be involved in the regulation of calcium channel function

        (3) May act as a glycine agonist

        (4) May increase effect of serotonin

        (5) May decrease kindling in neurons of the limbic system

    d. <u>Calcium channel blockers</u>

        (1) Prevent influx of calcium into neurons

        (2) Calcium is a major intracellular second messenger

4. **Side effects**

    a. <u>Lithium</u>

        (1) Sedation <u>not</u> common

       (2)   Fine hand tremor (treat with beta-blockers)

       (3)   Polyuria, polydipsia

       (4)   Leukocytosis

       (5)   Gastric irritation, nausea, diarrhea

       (6)   Hypothyroidism (in 10% of chronic patients) with or without goiter

       (7)   Weight gain

       (8)   Toxicity

          (a)   Confusion, coma

          (b)   Dysarthria, ataxia

          (c)   Hyperactive reflexes

          (d)   Cardiac abnormalities

b. <u>Anticonvulsants</u>

       (1)   Leukopenia

       (2)   Nausea, vomiting

       (3)   Dizziness, ataxia

       (4)   Sedation

       (5)   Hepatitis, aplastic anemia, agranulocytosis (rare, but serious)

c. <u>Calcium channel blockers</u>

       (1)   Hypotension

       (2)   Bradycardia

       (3)   Headache

       (4)   Dizziness

       (5)   Nausea

       (6)   Constipation

5. **Use in the Elderly**

   a. Side effects and toxicity occur at lower blood levels

   b. May be at increased risk for neurotoxicity

6. **Use in Pregnancy**

   a. Lithium and anticonvulsants are <u>very</u> teratogenic and <u>should not be used during pregnancy</u>

   b. Are secreted in breast milk

7. **Drug Interactions**

   a. All three classes of mood stabilizers interact with each other (increase or decrease blood levels) and increase risk of neurotoxicity, cardiotoxicity

   b. Concurrent use of antipsychotics may increase risk of neurotoxicity

   c. Many diuretics decrease lithium clearance and increase lithium levels

   d. Non-steroidal anti-inflammatory agents can increase lithium levels

8. **General Treatment Principles**

   a. Preliminary evaluation for lithium should include thyroid profile plus TSH, CBC, electrolytes, BUN/creatinine, EKG, pregnancy test

   b. Preliminary evaluation for anticonvulsants and calcium channel blockers should include CBC, liver profile, renal function studies

   c. Therapeutic blood levels important with lithium and anticonvulsants

      (1) Range for Lithium: 0.6 - 1.2 mEq/L

      (2) Range for Tegretol: 8 - 12 ug/ml

      (3) Range for Depakote: 40 - 150 mg/ml

   d. Lithium is mainstay drug; use alternatives if patient if non-responsive to lithium, a rapid cycler, history or evidence of brain damage and/or seizures

e. Hypothyroidism and renal toxicity can occur; measure thyroid and renal function every 6-12 months if maintenance therapy

E. <u>Antianxiety Agents/Sedative-Hypnotics</u> (anxiolytics, minor tranquilizers)

1. **Classes**

    a. <u>Benzodiazepines</u>

        (1)   Diazepam (Valium)

        (2)   Chlordiazepoxide (Librium)

        (3)   Lorazepam (Ativan)

        (4)   Alprazolam (Xanax)

        (5)   Oxazepam (Serax)

        (6)   Clorazepate (Tranxene)

        (7)   Prazepam (Centrax)

        (8)   Halazepam (Paxipam)

        (9)   Flurazepam (Dalmane)

        (10) Temazepam (Restoril)

        (11) Triazolam (Halcion)

        (12) Quazepam (Doral)

        (13) Clonazepam (Klonopin)

        (14) Midazolam (Versed)

    b. <u>Azaspirones</u>

        (1)   Buspirone (BuSpar)

    c. <u>Beta-blockers</u>

        (1)   Propranolol (Inderal)

        (2)   Metoprolol (Lopressor)

        (3)   Nadolol (Corgard)

        (4)   Atenolol (Tenormin)

    d. <u>Antihistamines</u>

       (1)   Hydroxyzine (Atarax, Vistaril)

       (2)   Diphenhydramine (Benadryl)

2. **Indications for use**

    a. <u>Generalized Anxiety Disorder</u>

    b. <u>Adjustment Disorder with Anxious Mood</u>

       (1)   Acute

    c. <u>Panic Disorder</u>

       (1)   Alprazolam, clonazepam

    d. <u>Social Phobia, Performance Anxiety</u>

       (1)   Beta-blockers

    e. <u>Alcohol withdrawal</u>

    f. <u>Acute psychotic state</u> (Schizophrenia, Mania, Catatonia, drug induced)

       (1)   Adjunct with antipsychotics

       (2)   Lorazepam: can be given IM

    g. <u>Seizure Disorders</u>

       (1)   Diazepam (IV) for status epilepticus.

    h. <u>Pre-op and pre-procedures</u>

       (1)   Lorazepam, diazepam

       (2)   Cause amnesia if given IV

       (3)   Reduces anxiety and relaxes muscles

    i. <u>Insomnia</u>

       (1)   Acute use only

       (2)   Reduces stage 3-4 or slow wave sleep and REM stage.

j. <u>Behavioral syndromes in mental retardation</u>: Buspar and Beta-blockers

   (1) Autistic symptoms

   (2) Hyperarousal

   (3) Aggression

   (4) Self injurious behavior

k. <u>Akathisia</u>

l. <u>Jet lag</u>: shift change problems.

3. **Mode of action**

   a. <u>Benzodiazepines</u>

      (1) Enhance activity of Gamma-Amino Butyric Acid (GABA).

      (2) Bind to benzodiazepine receptor (BZD).

      (3) BZD receptor and GABA receptor part of the same super-receptor complex with a chloride (Cl-) channel.

      (4) Increases Cl- ion flow into neuron and resulting hyperpolarization reduces the firing rate.

      (5) BZD receptors found in highest concentration in locus ceruleus (LC). Most norepinephrine neurons originate in LC.

   b. <u>Azaspirones (Buspar)</u>

      (1) Doesn't effect BZD or GABA receptors.

      (2) Agonist or partial agonist at serotonin (5-HT1A) receptors.

      (3) Blocks Dopamine (D_2) receptors (clinical effects unknown).

   c. <u>Beta-blockers</u>

      (1) Block norepinephrine (NE) and epinephrine (E) at the post-synaptic Beta-receptors (1 and 2).

d. <u>Antihistamines</u>

    (1)   Block histamine (H) receptors

    (2)   Also block muscarinic cholinergic receptors.

4. **Side Effects**

a. <u>Benzodiazepines</u>

    (1)   Sedation, decreased concentration, poor coordination, confusion.

    (2)   Paradoxical responses with rage, irritability, agitation-due to disinhibition.

    (3)   Anterograde amnesia-with short acting drugs at hypnotic doses.

    (4)   Exacerbation or precipitation of depression (except possibly Alprazolam).

    (5)   Tolerance to sedation but not to antianxiety effect.

    (6)   Physical dependence with subsequent withdrawal syndromes do occur (especially with high potency forms).

    (7)   Psychological dependence (habituation).

b. <u>Azaspirones</u>

    (1)   Nausea

    (2)   Dizziness

    (3)   Headache

    (4)   Nervousness

    (5)   Excitement

c. <u>Beta-blockers</u>

    (1)   Bradycardia

    (2)   Hypotension

    (3)   Sedation/fatigue

    (4)   Depression

        (5)   Contraindicated in asthma, diabetes, heart failure, COPD, hyperthyroidism

    d. <u>Antihistamines</u>

        (1)   Confusion, sedation, hypotension

        (2)   Anticholinergic effects

5. **Use in the Elderly**

    a. <u>Short half-life BZD's best</u>. To prevent accumulation and over-sedation.

    b. <u>Confusion</u> can be problematic

    c. May require <u>loser doses</u> for therapeutic effect.

    d. Buspar may be well tolerated.

6. **Use in Pregnancy**

    a. Avoid if possible.

    b. Are secreted in breast milk.

7. **Drug Interactions**

    a. Rate of elimination increased or decreased by a variety of drugs.

    b. Buspirone contraindicated with MAO inhibitors.

    c. Sedative effects additive with other CNS depressants.

    d. Cimetidine (Tagamet) increases blood levels of many benzodiazepines.

    e. Beta-blockers increase blood levels of antipsychotics.

F. <u>General Treatment Principles</u>

1. **Benzodiazepines**

    a. Drugs of choice for anxiety and insomnia.

    b. Low abuse potential if used appropriately.

    c. Long half-life drugs require hs or BID dosing.

    d. Short half-life drugs require TID or QID dosing.

e. Best <u>not</u> used in people with histories of substance abuse or some personality disorders (Borderline).

f. Long half-life drugs can accumulate over time.

g. Lorazepam and oxazepam have no active metabolite and do not accumulate.

h. Time limited use (not over 2-3 months).

i. Long-term use may be indicated in Panic Disorder.

j. Oral administration best. Lorazepam can be effective IM also.

k. Additive effects with alcohol.

l. Are all equally effective as anti-anxiety agents or hypnotics; differ in rate of onset, half-life, presence of active metabolite, potency.

m. <u>Should never be abruptly stopped</u>.

2. **Azaspirones (Buspar)**

a. Has no anticonvulsant, sedative or muscle relaxant effect.

b. Delayed onset of action (weeks).

c. Taken continuously, not PRN.

d. Not cross-tolerant with benzodiazepines.

e. Produces less cognitive impairment than BZD's.

f. Produces no dependence or withdrawal symptoms.

3. **Beta-blockers**

a. Differ in lipid-solubility and half-lives.

b. Differ in autonomic effects ($beta_1$ <u>versus</u> $beta_2$).

c. Best for peripheral symptoms of anxiety (tremors, tachycardia).

4. **Antihistamines**

a. May be used if co-existing skin disorders.

     b. Tolerance develops to sedative effects.

     c. Depresses REM sleep.

     d. Limited by anticholinergic side-effects.

III. SOMATIC THERAPIES

  A. <u>Electro-Convulsive Therapy (ECT)</u>

    1. **Types** (electrode placement)

      a. Unilateral - non-dominant side

      b. Bilateral

    2. **Indications for Use**

      a. <u>Major depression</u> especially with psychotic features.

      b. <u>Bipolar Disorder</u>, Depressed or Manic

      c. <u>Schizophrenia with catatonia</u>

      d. <u>Most useful</u> with:

        (1) Elderly with coexistent medical problems.

        (2) Acutely, actively suicidal patients.

        (3) Treatment resistant depression

    3. **Mode of Action**

      a. Bilateral generalized seizure necessary (35-60 seconds duration).

      b. Down-regulation of beta-adrenergic receptors after a series of treatments.

    4. **Side Effects**

      a. <u>Amnesia</u>

        (1) Anterograde and retrograde

        (2) After several treatments

        (3) Lasts weeks to months; rarely years.

(4) More common with bilateral mode, increased number of treatments.

b. Confusion

(1) Increases with increased number of treatments.

(2) Usually clears after treatments stop.

c. Fractures

(1) Rare now with adequate muscle relaxation medications.

d. Headaches

e. Bladder rupture

(1) Must empty bladder before treatment.

f. Brain herniation due to space occupying intracranial lesion.

g. Most complications due to general anesthesia, not ECT.

5. Use in the Elderly

a. Helpful if co-existing medical problems prevent use of medications.

b. Can be used with co-existing OBS.

c. Anesthesia risks most important.

6. Use in pregnancy

a. Safe if well ventilated.

b. May be safer than psychotropic drugs.

7. Contraindications

a. Increased intracranial pressure.

(1) ECT acutely increases CSF pressure.

(2) Herniation a risk

(3) Evaluate for papilledema

    b. Recent MI, significant arrhythmias, severe hypertension.

8. General Treatment Principles

    a. ECT is effective, safe and painless

    b. Mortality rate low, lower than meds or untreated disorder.

    c. There is a media/public relations problem.

    d. Informed consent from patient, relative, second psychiatrist.

    e. More effective (80%-90%) than antidepressant medication (70%).

    f. Usual protocol is one treatment per day, every other day (3/week).

    g. Usual number of treatments is 6-12 for depression and 10-20 for mania and Catatonic Schizophrenia.

    h. Improvement often seen after 1-6 treatments.

    i. Relapse rate high if not followed by maintenance medications.

    j. Unilateral produces less confusion and amnesia but more treatments required.

    k. Doesn't cure underlying disorder; interrupts acute episode.

9. Treatment Protocol

    a. Pre-treatment evaluation

        (1)   Complete history and physical especially cardiac and neurological.

        (2)   Complete lab evaluation including CBC, blood chemistry, UA, X-Ray of chest and spine, EKG.

        (3)   MRI, CT, EEG if needed.

    b. Treatment considerations.

        (1)   Empty bladder and bowels.

        (2)   NPO after MN

      (3)   Stop medications day before treatment

      (4)   Remove dentures; use bite block to protect teeth and tongue.

      (5)   CPR and ACLS capability necessary.

      (6)   Monitor EKG, EEG

      (7)   Anesthesiologist should be part of team.

c. <u>Medications</u>

      (1)   Atropine to control vagal arrhythmias and reduce secretions; may increase post-treatment confusion.

      (2)   100% O_2 by bag.

      (3)   Methohexital (Brevital) to produce a light anesthesia.

      (4)   Succinylcholine (Anectine) to paralyze muscles.

B. <u>Light Therapy</u>

1. **Types**

a. Phase advance: use lights to simulate dawn. Begun two hours before customary time for awakening.

b. Placing person in front of a screen emitting light five times brighter than ordinary room light for two hours each day.

c. Using a screen producing light 20 times brighter than normal room light for 30 minutes each day.

2. **Indications for Use**

a. Major Depression: Seasonal Affective Disorder (SAD)

b. Sleep-wake schedule disorder.

3. **Mode of Action**

a. Exposure to bright light in the **MORNING** results in a <u>phase advance</u> of biological rhythms.

b. <u>Delayed</u> circadian rhythms are associated with seasonal affective disorder.

      c. Full-spectrum light effective.

      d. Suprachiasmatic nucleus of hypothalamus thought to be the major endogenous pacemaker.

   4. **Side Effects**

      a. Irritability

      b. Headache

      c. Eye Strain

   5. **General Treatment Principles**

      a. Bright light necessary (2500 lux).

      b. 2-3 hours every day in the MORNING.

      c. Direct viewing not needed; periodic glances at light sufficient.

      d. Response seen often after 2-4 days of treatment.

      e. Relapse seen 2-4 days after treatment stops.

C. Stereotactic psychosurgery is being applied to chronic intractable mental disorders which have demonstrated neurologic loci (e.g., Obsessive Compulsive Disorders, OCD).

IV. MAJOR INDIVIDUAL INTERPERSONAL TREATMENT MODALITIES

Prognosis is best when the patient has a strong ego, a stable environment, adequate intelligence, and has temporarily decompensated under overwhelming stress.

A. Behavior Modification

   1. **Behavior modification therapies** are based on psychological principles.

      a. Reinforcement: Identification of the appropriate reinforcer is a central issue.

      b. Learning and relearning, is the basis of all Behavior Modification therapies.

      c. Anxiety gradient: relationship between the nearness to a feared object and the height of the anxiety.

d. IMPORTANT NOTE: Focus is to <u>change symptoms</u>. Success rate for target symptoms: generally the upper 90%.

2. **Different Behavior Modification Therapies**

   a. <u>Operant Conditioning</u> (Skinner)

   (1)   Basic principle is to reward an appropriate behavior and, over time, that behavior will repeat. Or remove something the person likes (e.g., attention) and the behavior will disappear or extinguish.

   (2)   The principle for <u>shaping behavior</u>. E.g., in the treatment of autism, the child is food deprived and each time he makes a sound he is given something to eat. At first, any sound will do; later on, the child only gets food for producing words and sentences.

   (3)   <u>Token economy systems</u>: focus is on developing social behavior. Can earn tokens towards something they desire (weekend pass) if they produce certain types of behaviors. At first, any behavior will do, but later, the behavior must be more socialized to get the token.

   (4)   Pain control as an example.

       (a)   Pain is influenced by: <u>ethnicity</u>; <u>symbolic meaning</u>, e.g. "I'm not a man"; and <u>learning</u>: therefore, chronic pain can persist after organic reasons are gone.

       (b)   Can attenuate by: <u>no reinforcement</u> (remove attention); <u>relaxation</u>; <u>biofeedback</u>; <u>hypnosis</u>

   (5)   IMPORTANT NOTE: simply assessing a behavior (counting its frequency, measuring its size, etc.) will lead to a decrease in the behavior.

   b. <u>Aversive Therapy</u>

   (1)   Applications:

       (a)   Alcoholics who take antabuse

       (b)   "Junk food addict": person views picture of favorite "junk" food and is shocked while looking. Shock is stopped when the person presses a button that replaces the original picture with a more wholesome food.

    (c)   Enuresis: the patient is not routinely shocked; but rather, wetting the bed completes a circuit which turns on a light or bell. Consequently, the child in sleep learns to recognize the pressure of urine building up in the bladder and awakens.

c. Desensitization: The person is encouraged to interact with the frightening objects or ideas until they are successful or until that particular idea or object no longer provokes anxiety, e.g. stage fright; the person is placed in a similar situation and forced to speak to an audience.

d. Systematic desensitization variant of the desensitization procedure. (WOLPE)

    (1)   First a hierarchy of parts of the feared situation is established. Then, the person is taught to relax.

    (2)   After he has relaxed, the person visualizes the lowest item on the hierarchical list. If no anxiety appears, proceeds to the next step in the hierarchy. If anxiety appears, imagery is stopped and person re-relaxes.

    (3)   Person is relaxed and uses visual imagery only. Anxiety is not allowed to appear.

    (4)   The hypothesis is that relaxation and anxiety cannot occur simultaneously. If you keep the person relaxed during the imagery, they cannot attach anxiety to the mental representation.

3. **Flooding therapies:** Same as desensitization but uses imagery not the real feared object.

4. **Biofeedback**

a. Biofeedback: a biological or physiologic process of which the persons are not normally aware is fed back to them (e.g., by turning on a light) and they are requested to continue keeping that physiological or biological process going by maintaining the feedback signal.

b. Alpha waves and theta waves of the EEG; and the EMG of the frontalis muscle have been used.

    c. Typically, what is fed back to the person is a biological or physiological process that is incompatible with a particular symptom. E.g., being in the EEG Alpha state is incompatible with anxiety. Also, the frontalis and occipital muscles being relaxed are incompatible with tension headaches.

    d. Biofeedback has been utilized to teach epileptic patients to abort seizures; to teach people to raise the temperature of their skin by vasodilation which can attenuate migraine headaches. Other applications have been to decrease blood pressure, reduced stomach acidity, etc..

B. Individual Interpersonal Psychotherapies

  1. In traditional psychotherapy therapists are treating the psychodynamic psychological processes within the individual and how these interact with the family, his small group, and the community.

  2. In psychological therapies, the relationship between the therapist and the patient is emphasized. The therapist is doing something with the patient, not to him (in contrast to the Behavior Modification therapies, which imply doing something to the patient).

  3. Three important elements to all psychotherapies: talking freely to someone who is relatively non-critical; catharsis or "blowing off steam"; desensitization - simply by going over something, it is less disturbing. Additionally,

    a. Clarification: as one hears oneself talk about a problem, it may be understood differently.

    b. Abreaction: as a person talks about something, he often releases "repressed" feelings which may vent in the session. Once these are "vented", they no longer are a source of conflict.

  4. Important elements about the therapy: patient may feel he is **not alone**; that he **can be understood**; and he is **not hopeless**.

    a. Corrective emotional experience: the patient may go through some difficulties with the therapist that caused trouble before, but that he now understands differently.

    b. Termination: the therapist must terminate the therapy in such a way that there is a final clear, healthy termination of the relationship between the patient and the therapist.

5. **Specific therapeutic undertakings by the therapist:**

   a. <u>Interpretation</u>: helping the patient make sense out of what is going on so that the patient can assume some control. Often reinterpreting presumed motivations for others' actions.

   b. <u>Therapist attitudes</u>: the therapist must become congruent with himself and expect people to get well. The therapist who is nurturant is a much more curative factor than the types of therapeutic methods (TA, Gestalt, etc.) used by the therapist. Apparently, <u>over time</u>, therapists who come from different philosophical or theoretical schools look more alike in what they do than they look different.

6. **Classical psychoanalysis:** requires many years for completion (approximately 3-10). <u>It works best with persons who are not psychotic and are distressed by their symptoms</u>.

   a. Aim is to make unconscious material conscious. Focuses on dream interpretation, transference issues, and insight. Strengthens the Ego. "Where Id is there shall Ego be."

   b. The assumption is that if the pathogenic unconscious becomes conscious, the patient can understand and control symptoms.

   c. Resistance is the same as defense mechanisms. As resistance is overcome (defenses are broken down), the patient develops a "transference neurosis" to the therapist which is "worked through."

   d. <u>Free Association</u> (saying the first thing that comes into awareness without any censoring) and analysis of dreams are the principle methods of psychoanalysis in getting to unconscious material that "needs to be made conscious."

   e. <u>Transference Neurosis</u>: The patient projects on the analyst (re-experiences distorted feelings, etc.,) from the past as if they are happening again, leading to an exacerbation of the conflict within the hour. Skillful interpretation by the analyst allows working through of the transference.

f. Psychoanalysis has been adapted to treating psychotic individuals, but this treatment is extremely time consuming and therefore expensive.

7. **Psychoanalytically oriented psychotherapy:**

   a. Aimed towards restructuring the basic psychodynamics and personality of the individual person.

   b. These proceed from a common assumption that unless a child is born brain damaged or autistic, the child develops disorders as a reaction to the environment and parents. Probably somewhere around the ages of 7-9 years old, this reaction becomes internalized; therefore, changing the environment or the parents will not matter a great deal.

   c. Rogerian therapy's basic orientation is that the therapist assumes an unconditional positive regard for the patient in the context of a warm, accepting, and understanding environment; coupled with reflecting the patient's statement in a non-evaluative way the patient will have a corrective emotional experience and be less debilitated.

   d. Transactional Analysis as a therapy <u>focuses on understanding</u> the transactions among one's own Ego States; and between one's and other's Ego States which reinforce pathologic life scripts. <u>Useful to help people think before they act.</u>

   e. Gestalt therapy, on the other hand, is grounded in Gestalt psychology theory. In Gestalt therapy the focus is on the figure ground reversals in the person's perceptions and closure of uncompleted Gestalts. <u>Gestalt focuses on internal feelings--not words</u>. <u>Useful to help people feel</u>.

      (1) In Gestalt it is assumed that patients "scare themselves" by:

         (a) What they do with their breathing: usually they hold their breath.

         (b) The strength of inhalation: they either hyperventilate or hypoventilate.

         (c) They get out of the here and now and begin to imagine future catastrophes (catastrophic expectations).

8. **Cognitive Behavioral**

   a. Focus is to correct automatic thoughts which are self-deprecatory and self-defeating in nature.

   b. Underlying assumption is that cognitions (thoughts) control feelings or emotions. One must change the thoughts to change the feelings.

   c. The behavioral component emphasizes that the person must actively do something in order to change. E.g., if the person is depressed and staying in bed all day, they must get out of bed each day. Behavioral patterns are gradually increased to a more adaptive life style.

9. **Supportive Psychotherapy**: This is sometimes called brief psychotherapy. The techniques that are especially valuable in brief psychotherapy are:

   a. Active interpretation of reality

   b. Ventilation, catharsis, or abreaction in a supportive atmosphere

   c. Suggestion, persuasion, or direction

   d. Re-education

   e. Installation of a sense of hope and optimism

V. **GROUP METHODS**

A. <u>Group Treatment</u>:

   1. There is one therapist with many patients. The therapist is clearly defined and his role can be to direct and clarify the therapeutic interactions among and between the various patients. Interactions can be very confrontational of the patient's self destructive behavior.

   2. Group treatment can be of any specific theory orientations; that is, TA, Gestalt, Psychoanalytic, etc..

   3. Group treatment offers the advantages of therapy in the context of group support and confrontation. Allows the patient to try out new behaviors in a supportive and

nonthreatening environment. Also sees in others, the difficulties is having with self.

B. Group Process:

1. Here there is no designated therapist. The process between the persons in the group is examined.

2. It is the role of group facilitators to point out the interactions in the group, but they are not therapists. This is not treatment.

C. Family Therapy: Because of the assumption that the family is frequently the etiology of a person's disturbance, treatment has begun to focus on the family as a whole. This is a special form of a combination of group therapy and group process. The following are important aspects of Family Therapy:

1. **A family is a system:** All systems have three common characteristics.

a. External boundaries: We can fight like hell among ourselves but no one else (e.g., physician) can say anything bad about us.

b. Internal maintenance: Types of feelings allowed to go on within the family system. E.g., it is OK to fight and hate one another, but it is not OK to love.

c. Roles: Can be either verbal or non-verbal. Define e.g., the roles of big people vs. the roles of little people.

(1) **Indicated patient:** in a disturbed family situation, there is one person who is, by common agreement of the family, the "indicated patient." That person manifests psychopathological traits on behalf of the family.

(2) **Role stability:** In "sick families" there may be very stable roles in the family, e.g. blamer, placator, irrelevant, intellectualizer; but the person who fills each role may switch. (Virginia Satir).

(3) If the indicated patient is treated outside the family and "gets well," someone else in the family may fill the patient role.

    (4)   Usually, when a family comes to a therapist requesting a change, what they mean is that they want the family to go back to what it was before the children began to have sexual urges, rebellious aggressive urges, etc.

VI.   ENVIRONMENTAL MANIPULATIONS

A. Milieu Therapy: The assumption is that "if the environment can drive a person crazy, it can also drive them sane". The structure of the environment is used to set boundaries, limitations, and to define the world as safe for the patient. Most therapeutic endeavors with persons who have psychotic level disturbance are milieu therapy oriented.

1. Short term inpatient hospitalization

   a. Brief stay: 1-2 weeks

   b. Person has had an acute onset of severe problems

   c. Focus on relief from stressors (protection)

   d. Diagnostic workup

   e. Medication stabilization

   f. Other somatic stabilization

2. Day hospital

   a. Continuum of care from short term inpatient hospitalization.

   b. Indications: person who has had acute short term inpatient hospitalization; or a patient who doesn't need total inpatient care.

   c. Is really outpatient care; however patient is present in the facility from 1/2 to full day; 3-5 days per week.

   d. Does not sleep over in the facility.

   e. Patient usually attends for a few months.

   f. Often a transition to outpatient, once/week, psychotherapy.

3. **Day treatment**

   a. Non-residential expanded care; usually for
      chronically mentally ill persons.

   b. Spends major portion of their day in this facility.

   c. Does not sleep over in the facility.

   d. May have a sheltered workshop associated where
      patients can earn money.

   e. Patients usually stay with these facilities for
      years.

4. **Long term**

   a. Not common today. Some custodial facilities still
      exist; however, most chronic care patients are in
      other settings.

   b. Where they exist the patient is in the facility for
      years; and in some cases, as in domiciliaries, are
      never expected to leave.

   c. Care is mainly custodial and supportive.

   d. Very little demand for productivity is made on the
      patients.

5. **Therapeutic Communities:** In therapeutic communities,
   there is an agreement between patients and staff that
   patients have a significant voice in the management of
   the unit, as well as the management of other patients.
   For instance, the patient group as a whole may recommend
   that a particular patient's medication be increased or
   decreased.

   a. Usually these are facilities that are addressing a
      self destructive **life style**, e.g., chemical
      dependence. Usually not dealing with psychotically
      disturbed individuals.

   b. Highly structured with a strong work ethic to
      progressively earn more freedom of action and status
      in the community.

c. <u>NOTE</u>:   In Milieu Therapy as well as Therapeutic Community facilities, if one finds patients acting out (fighting, having sexual relations on the unit, running away from the institution, committing suicide), entertain two possibilities:

   (1)   Patient behavior is reflecting staff behavior (members of the staff are fighting or they are having affairs (either "fighting or fucking").

   (2)   A new patient has been admitted who is serving as a role model for the behavior. That is, there is a contagion phenomenon where one patient has seen another patient do the act and imitates.

B. <u>Community Mental Health Centers (CMHCS)</u>:   Have been part of the Public Mental Health System. Traditionally supported in part by federal monies to State Mental Health Departments and a sliding scale patient fee system.

1. There are 12 services which CMHCS offer.   These are: inpatient services, outpatient services, partial hospitalization, 24-hour emergency psychiatric service, consultation, education to the community, court screening, transitional living facility, special services for children, special services for elderly, programs for alcoholics, and programs for drug dependent persons.   Research and evaluation of services delivery are also required if Federal Funding helps support the CMHC.

2. Major focus is a continuity of care so a given person can enter at an Inpatient Unit, be released to a transitional living facility or a more outpatient program (and vice-versa); yet still be within the same health care delivery system.

3. Usually requires a Board of Directors with which representatives of the community, the political system, and the consumer populations are involved.

4. Operate in a given catchment area so treatment can be effected close to the home of the patient.

CHAPTER 4

ORGANIC BRAIN CONDITIONS

I. **BACKGROUND**

   A. <u>Definition</u>

      1. Disorders of behavior and mental functioning caused by organic brain pathology (damage or dysfunction). Underlying disorder may be primary (intracerebral) or secondary (extracerebral).

      2. Characteristics, course and treatment are dependent upon the nature, severity, cause, and location of the underlying organic disorder.

   B. <u>General Observations</u>

      1. It was originally thought that any etiological factor affecting the brain would cause a specific, distinctive disease with a consistent set of symptoms.

      2. Later, the pendulum swung into the opposite extreme and it was commonly held that from a pathophysiological point of view the brain had only one mode of response irrespective of type, extent or localization of the damaging agent. Differences were merely due to intensity of the brain reaction (psychotic vs. non-psychotic) and to duration (reversible - acute; permanent = chronic).

      3. The truth is probably in the middle. From an empirical clinical point of view, it is possible to distinguish several separate "brain diseases", but they share many common characteristics.

         a. First, most organic mental diseases are characterized by a disturbance of self-awareness (orientation, if in the present; and memory, if in the past).

         b. Second, they usually affect higher intellectual function, judgement, cognition, and emotional control.

         c. Third, there is only a very loose and unreliable correlation between the nature, the location, and the extent of the damaging process and the ensuing disease picture.

         d. Fourth, the rate and speed with which the disease develops appears important.

e. Fifth, and most important, the premorbid personality
of the patient will decisively influence the disease
picture, either by the unmasking of previously
repressed and latent traits, or by the defensive
exaggeration of personality characteristics.

C. Etiologies: The Mnemonic MITTEN,CDV is helpful in
understanding the causes of organic brain conditions.

1. Metabolic

2. Infection

3. Trauma

4. Toxin

5. Endocrine

6. Neoplastic

7. Congenital

8. Degenerative

9. Vascular

II. **CLASSIFICATION OF ORGANIC MENTAL SYNDROMES (IRRESPECTIVE OF ETIOLOGY)**

A. NOTE:

1. Organic Mental **Disorder** = known etiology.

2. Organic Mental **Syndromes** = unknown etiology.

B. Global cognitive impairment

1. Dementia - pervasive intellectual decline in the face of a clear sensorium.

2. Delirium - fluctuating levels of arousal

C. Selective cognitive impairment

1. Amnestic syndrome

2. Organic hallucinosis

D. Predominately manifested by <u>personality disturbance</u> or resemblance to "functional" mental disorders.

1. Organic anxiety syndrome

2. Organic mood syndrome

3. Organic delusional syndrome

4. Organic personality syndrome

E. Associated with ingestion or reduction in the use of a substance

1. **Intoxication**

2. **Withdrawal**

III. **DISORDERS OF GLOBAL COGNITIVE FUNCTIONING**

A. <u>Dementia</u>

1. **Symptoms**

a. <u>Prodromal</u>

(1)   Subtle personality changes

(2)   Decrease in interests and enthusiasm

(3)   Labile and shallow affect

(4)   Agitation

(5)   Physical/psychiatric complaints

(6)   Gradual loss of intellectual skills

(7)   Depression

b. <u>Manifest</u>

(1)   USUALLY <u>NO</u> CLOUDING OF CONSCIOUSNESS

(2)   Memory loss (often with confabulation)

(3)   Changes in mood and personality

(4)   Loss of orientation

(5)   Intellectual impairment

     (6)   Impaired judgement

     (7)   Psychotic symptoms

     (8)   Language impairment

     (9)   Impaired social and/or occupational functioning

2. **Etiology** - Due to widespread cerebral dysfunction, but <u>Not</u> a diagnosis by itself

   a. "<u>Untreatable</u>"

     (1)   Primary degeneration (Alzheimers' Disease) - most common form of dementia. Posterior brain disease: see dysfunction in Temporal-Parietal areas. Locus ceruleus loss. Question of pathology in Beta-amyloid production. Probably pathology begins in cortex and results in retrograde axonal degeneration. Probably a multi-neurotransmitter disease.

     (2)   Huntington's Chorea

     (3)   Parkinson's Disease

   b. "<u>Treatable</u>" causes

     (1)   Multi-infarct - second most common form of dementia

     (2)   Normal pressure hydrocephalus

     (3)   Alcohol

     (4)   Other drugs

     (5)   Tumors

     (6)   Trauma

     (7)   Infection

     (8)   Metabolic disorders

     (9)   Heart, lung, kidney, liver disease

c. <u>AIDS</u>

    (1)   Direct HIV infection of CNS

    (2)   Intracranial tumors and infections due to immune impairment

    (3)   Indirect effects of systemic disease

d. <u>Psychosocial factors</u>

    (1)   Premorbid personality, intelligence, education

    (2)   Rapidity of onset

    (3)   Current emotional state

3. **Course:**   3 courses depending on cause

a. <u>Gradual</u> (e.g., primary degenerative dementia)

b. <u>Sudden</u> (e.g., head trauma)

c. <u>Stepwise</u> (e.g., multi-infarct dementia)

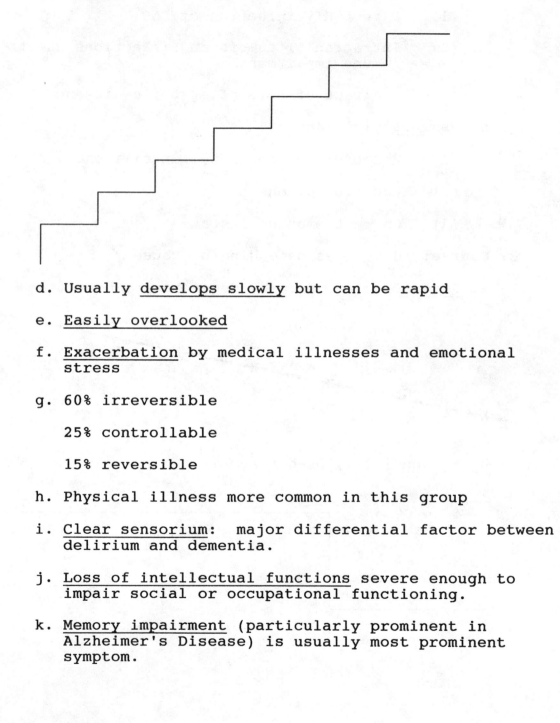

d. Usually <u>develops slowly</u> but can be rapid

e. <u>Easily overlooked</u>

f. <u>Exacerbation</u> by medical illnesses and emotional stress

g. 60% irreversible

   25% controllable

   15% reversible

h. Physical illness more common in this group

i. <u>Clear sensorium</u>: major differential factor between delirium and dementia.

j. <u>Loss of intellectual functions</u> severe enough to impair social or occupational functioning.

k. <u>Memory impairment</u> (particularly prominent in Alzheimer's Disease) is usually most prominent symptom.

1. <u>One of following four</u>:

    (1)   Impaired abstract thinking;

    (2)   Impaired judgement;

    (3)   Impaired other higher cortical functions (e.g. aphasia);

    (4)   Personality change.

m. <u>Evidence of organic, physical factor</u> or no functional disorder.

n. Generally <u>slow and progressive</u> with time.

o. <u>Pseudodementia</u> is Major Depressive Disorder often confused with dementia in older people.

B. <u>Delirium</u>

1. **Other names:** Acute brain syndrome, toxic psychosis, metabolic encephalopathy) Common - 10-15% of all acute medical inpatients.

    a. <u>Two essential features</u>:

        (1)   Reduced ability to maintain attention to external stimuli and/or ability to shift attention to a new stimulus.

        (2)   Disorganized thinking: rambling, irrelevant or incoherent speech.

    b. <u>Symptoms</u>

        (1)   **Prodromal**

            (a)   Restlessness, anxiety

            (b)   Insomnia

            (c)   Vivid dreams and nightmares

            (d)   Hypersensitivity to light and sound

            (e)   Fleeting illusions and hallucinations

(f) Distractibility

(g) Difficulty thinking clearly

(2) **Manifest**

(a) **CLOUDING OF CONSCIOUSNESS: LEVEL OF
CONSCIOUSNESS IS REDUCED**

(b) <u>Develops rapidly and fluctuates with time</u>

(c) Attention deficit

(d) Perceptual disturbances: hallucinations and
illusions

(e) Sleep - wake alteration

(f) Disorientation

(g) Memory impairment

(h) Incoherence

(i) Altered psychomotor activity

(j) Often emotional features accompany delirium
(exaggerated display of any emotion)

(3) **Resolution**

(a) Usually lasts less than a week

(b) Stepwise resolution

(c) Often worse at night

(d) Final outcome:

- complete resolution - most common

- lasting residual impairment (dementia)

- death

2. Etiology

   a. Multifactorial

   b. Widespread derangement of cerebral metabolism rather than local lesions; dysfunction of cerebral cortex and certain subcortical structures.

   c. Cerebral

   d. Systemic

   e. Differentiate from acute "functional" psychosis.

IV. DISORDERS OF SELECTIVE COGNITIVE IMPAIRMENT

A. Amnestic Syndrome

1. Those symptoms that signal the diagnosis are the impairment of short term and recent (last decade) memory; while remote memory or overlearned material is unaffected.

2. Etiology includes a wide variety of toxic, infectious, structural, and traumatic events.

3. Course and treatment is dependent upon the etiologic condition and whether it can be brought under control.

B. Organic Hallucinosis

1. Central to this diagnostic entity are hallucinations in one or more sensory modality. They may be persistent or episodic.

2. Etiology again can be a variety of toxic, structural, or infectious processes.

3. Course and treatment is dependent upon the etiology.

V. DISORDERS OF ORGANIC PERSONALITY DISTURBANCE

A. Caveat: because these disorders can mimic established "functional" disorders, it is imperative that persons who have a sudden onset of behavior that is "abnormal" be carefully worked up from a medical standpoint.

B. **Organic Anxiety Syndrome/Disorder**

1. Definition: anxiety and/or panic attacks that are recurrent and have no psychodynamic "meaning".

2. Etiology is an established organic condition: e.g., metabolic, endocrine, toxic, cardio-vascular, etc., dysfunctions.

3. Course and treatment is dependent upon the etiology.

4. NOTE: in this condition, because anxiety symptoms are so disruptive for the person, a secondary cognitive impairment (e.g., distractibility, poor concentration) may appear. Usually remits when the pathologic condition is successfully addressed.

C. **Organic Mood Syndrome/Disorder**

1. Definition: manic or depressed moods that accompany a clearly organic condition.

2. Etiology is most frequently toxicity, medication side effects, endocrine complications, infections, structural lesions, etc..

3. Course and treatment is dependent upon the etiology.

4. Because of the predominant mood associations, suicide and sometimes homicide are accompaniments of this Syndrome/Disorder.

D. **Organic Delusional Syndrome/Disorder**

1. Definition: false fixed belief systems (delusion) that occur in a state of full consciousness, which are the result of an organic condition.

2. Etiology: most common in America is substance abuse. Also reported with temporal lobe lesions and some degenerative diseases.

3. Course and treatment is dependent upon the etiology.

E. <u>Organic Personality Syndrome/Disorder</u>

   1. Definition: a clear change in personality style and traits, which are associated with an organic condition. May be the accentuation of a previous trait or personality variable. May be social inappropriateness, aggressiveness, etc.

   2. Occurs in a clear level of consciousness.

   3. Etiology: most common is a traumatic head injury although structural changes and toxic conditions can cause the condition.

   4. Course and treatment is dependent upon the etiology.

VI. **DISORDERS ASSOCIATED WITH INGESTION OR REDUCTION IN THE USE OF A SUBSTANCE**

See Chapter 5, Substance Abuse Disorders.

SUBSTANCE ABUSE

I. **DEFINITIONS**

   A. <u>Addiction (Abuse and Dependence)</u>: a state of periodic or chronic intoxication, detrimental to the individual and/or society, caused by repeated consumption of a drug with the characteristics of:

      1. **Habituation**: psychological dependence or taking out of habit.

      2. **Tolerance**: decreased effect with repeated doses of the same dose level of the drug.

      3. **Dependence**: physiological response to the abrupt termination of drug leads to observable <u>physical</u> signs.

   B. <u>Alcoholism</u>

      1. Does not have self-control regarding the use of alcoholic beverages. Once starts drinking has great difficulty stopping. After the person has taken the first drink there is virtually no control.

      2. Dysfunction in one or more of five areas.

         a. Marital/familial - X7 separation/divorce rate of general population.

            (1)   Incest (44%)

            (2)   Spouse abuse (48%)

            (3)   Problems for the children

         b. Social (isolation):

            (1)   Friends stop inviting the person to social functions;

            (2)   Progressively isolates self to socialize only with persons who drink more and more.

         c. Occupational:

            (1)   On the job accidents;

            (2)   Chronically late for work;

            (3)   Shifts job frequently.

d. Legal:

    (1)   Legal intoxication: 100-150 mgm% B.A.L. (D.U.I.)

    (2)   Debts, alimony, accidents, etc.

e. Physical/Psychological (most common observed signs and symptoms)

    (1)   **Blackouts:** after consuming alcohol, carries on normal appearing behavior; however, no recall later on. Not a diagnosis in and of itself.

    (2)   Chronic gastritis: ulcers, etc.

    (3)   Cirrhosis: 14% of alcoholics die from this.

    (4)   Nutritional disorders: Pellagra, Beriberi, vitamin deficiency.

    (5)   Cancer, particularly of upper alimentary canal and bladder.

    (6)   Esophageal varices.

    (7)   Hypertension.

    (8)   Hypoglycemia.

    (9)   Depression.

    (10)   Sleep problems.

    (11)   Alcoholic hepatitis.

    (12)   Pancreatitis in absence of cholelithiasis.

C. "Teenage alcoholic"

Same diagnostic signs as for the adult don't apply exactly. Diagnosis includes having been drunk at least six times during the year; AND having trouble with:

1. **Family:** little involvement; argumentative.

2. **Social** (friends): only involved with persons who drink.

3. **School:** grades and decorum deteriorate.

4. **Legal:** stealing, traffic violations.

5. **Physical:** Gastrointestinal distress, sleep problems.

6. **Behavioral dysfunction:** oppositional, disruptive.

D. <u>Social drinker</u>: Drinks as much as associates. Not to excess, and only on social occasions. "Some people are more social than others."

E. <u>Problem drinker</u>: Problems for self and society. <u>Can</u> stop if problems are brought to attention.

II. **MAJOR PSYCHIATRIC DIAGNOSTIC CATEGORIES**

A. <u>Alcohol Organic Mental Disorders</u>

1. **Alcohol intoxication**

a. Recent ingestion of alcohol.

b. Maladaptive behavioral changes: e.g., disinhibition of sexual or aggressive impulses, mood lability, impaired judgement, impaired social or occupational functioning.

c. A physical sign of slurred speech, incoordination, unsteady gait, nystagmus, and/or flushed face.

2. **Alcohol idiosyncratic reaction**

a. Atypical aggressive or assaultive behavior, occurring within minutes of ingesting an amount of alcohol insufficient to induce intoxication in most people.

3. **Uncomplicated alcohol withdrawal**

a. Cessation of prolonged heavy drinking; OR, reduction in the amount consumed. This is followed, within several hours, by coarse tremor of hands, tongue, or eyelids.

b. Accompanied by: nausea and vomiting; malaise or weakness; autonomic hyperactivity (tachycardia, sweating, high BP); anxiety; depressed mood or irritability;transient hallucinations or illusions; headache; or insomnia.

4. **Alcohol withdrawal delirium**

a. Delirium (usually within one week post reduction or cessation) with a clouding of consciousness.

  b. Clinical features of delirium develop over a short period of time and tend to fluctuate over the course of the day.

 5. **Alcohol hallucinosis**

  a. Vivid auditory (sometime visual) hallucinations usually within 48 hours of stopping or reducing intake. The patient responds to the hallucinations with appropriate content.

  b. This occurs in the context of clear consciousness.

 6. **Alcohol amnestic disorder:** Short and long term memory loss. Not due to delirium or dementia. Follows prolonged heavy ingestion of alcohol.

 7. **Dementia associated with alcoholism:** dementia following prolonged heavy ingestion of alcohol; and persisting at least 3 weeks after cessation of alcohol ingestion.

B. <u>Psychoactive Substance Disorders.</u> The specific substance disorder diagnosis is dependent upon which substance the person has ingested.

 1. **Abuse**

  a. A maladaptive pattern of psychoactive substance use reflected by one or more of the following:

   (1) Continued use despite knowledge of having a persistent or recurrent social, occupational, psychological, or physical problem that is caused or exacerbated by use of the psychoactive substance.

   (2) Recurrent use in situations in which it is physically hazardous (e.g., driving while intoxicated).

  b. Some symptoms of the disturbance have been present for at least one month, or have occurred repeatedly over a longer period of time.

 2. **Dependence:** At least three of the following:

  a. Substance often taken in larger amounts or over a longer period than the person intended. Some symptoms of the disturbance have been present for at least one month, or have occurred repeatedly over a long period of time.

b. Persistent desire for the drug; or, one or more unsuccessful efforts to cut down or control substance use.

c. A great deal of time spent in activities necessary to get the substance (e.g., theft, looking for a dealer), taking the substance (e.g., chain smoking, I.V. injection) or recovering from its effects (e.g., hangover).

d. Frequent intoxication or withdrawal symptoms when expected to fulfill major role obligations at work, school, or home (e.g., does not go to work because hung over, goes to school or work "high", intoxicated while taking care of his or her children), or when substance use is physically hazardous (e.g., drives when intoxicated).

e. Important social, occupational, or recreational activities given up or reduced because of substance abuse. Withdraws from non-drug related social activities.

f. Continued substance use despite knowledge of having a persistent or recurrent social, psychological, or physical problem that is caused or exacerbated by the use of the substance (e.g., keeps using heroin despite family arguments about it, cocaine-induced depression, or having an ulcer made worse by using L.S.D. containing strychnine).

g. Marked tolerance; need for markedly increased amounts of the substance (i.e., at least a 50% increase) in order to achieve intoxication or desired effect, or markedly diminished effect with continued use of the same amount.

NOTE: The following items may not apply to cannabis, hallucinogens, or phencyclidine (PCP) dependence:

h. Characteristic withdrawal symptoms

i. Substance often taken to relieve or avoid withdrawal symptoms.

3. **Dual Disorder or Co-morbidity:** A recent term applied to those persons who have a diagnosable Substance Abuse Disorder, **AND** an additional other psychiatric disorder, e.g., Schizophrenia.

a. Approximately 50% of substance abusing/dependent persons have an additional disorder.

b. The most common co-morbid diagnosis is Antisocial Personality Disorder; however, all other psychiatric disorders are represented.

c. Frequently the chemical dependence is an attempt by the person to self medicate the underlying psychiatric disturbance.

d. One must treat both the Substance Abuse Disorder and the Psychiatric Disorder simultaneously.

e. An additional issue of co-morbidity is that of HIV+/AIDS.

   (1) Intravenous drug users often inoculate themselves with the HIV.

   (2) Drug users are also susceptible to this disease because the effects of the drugs often decrease inhibition regarding involvement in higher risk sexual activity.

III. **INTERVENTION**

A. General Issues in Treatment

1. Because **denial** of the disease is central to the disease itself, getting a person into treatment is difficult. The person denies that he has a problem. E.g., "I'm not an alcoholic. I just like the effects of alcohol. I can stop any time that I want, I just don't want to stop."

2. "Intervention" is a concept which involves the significant others (e.g., spouse, employer, parents, children, friends, etc.) of the drug dependent person gathering together with the person; and, confronting that person with the negative behavioral effects of the person's drug use. Person is usually given options: e.g., "get help or get out".

3. **Employee Assistance Programs (EAP):** Programs funded by an employer which offers assistance to the individual who is having problems with substance abuse and other mental health problems. They tend to have high rates of success secondary to potential job threat if the person doesn't take the referral made by the EAP person. Very cost effective. "The most expressive thing to do with a substance abuser is to fire them.

B. <u>Treatment of chemical dependence (includes alcoholism)</u>:

PROGRAM STRUCTURE IS SIMILAR REGARDLESS OF THE DRUG ABUSED.

1. **Three stages of treatment:** Each stage takes about 2 years to complete.

    a. <u>Withdrawal and abstinence</u>

        (1)   Medical management: titrated withdrawal often with cross dependent drug (e.g. benzodiazepines for alcoholism); nutritional needs; close observation; warm supportive environment.

        (2)   Abstinence: After withdrawal the focus is on not taking the first drink or the first drug.

    b. <u>Stress Coping</u>: focus is on learning to cope with everyday life without the chemical coping mechanisms of drugs.

    c. <u>Intrapersonal relations</u>: emphasis is on establishing new non-chemical based relationships with others.

C. <u>Comparative Therapeutic Modalities</u>

	Crisis Intervention	Therapeutic Community	Chemical Blockade
Inpatient			
Intermediate			
Outpatient			

1. **Inpatient, Intermediate and Outpatient care**

    a. <u>Inpatient</u>: Maximum environmental control.

    b. <u>Intermediate Care</u>: the person lives in a structured environment for a portion of the time: e.g., Half-Way House, but carries on regular activities the remaining time.

c. <u>Outpatient</u>: Latter stages or person has a strong, protective, positive support system.

2. **Crisis Intervention**: e.g., emergency rooms, social detoxification centers, etc.. Focus is only on detoxification, not rehabilitation.

3. **Therapeutic Community (TC)**

   a. <u>Inpatient (TC)</u>: long term, self supporting, live-in facilities.

   b. <u>Intermediate care (TC)</u>: person lives in a half-way house. Spends much of the 24 hour day working, at home taking care of family; however, that portion of the day where there is high risk of relapse is spent in the intermediate care facility. Here there is maximum support for abstinence and "destructive life style" change.

   c. <u>Outpatient (TC)</u>: long term association with an identified program usually of a "self help" variety.

      (1) Alcoholics Anonymous (AA): Self help program with no charge associated. Includes abstinence, introspection, public admission of alcoholism, and meeting dependency needs. Organized "12-step" program.

      (2) Narcotics Anonymous (NA): similar to AA except more specifically directed towards persons who have abused narcotics.

   d. <u>Issues of the Therapeutic Community</u>:

      (1) Less expensive

      (2) Positive atmosphere

      (3) Continuity of care

      (4) Decreased use of the expensive medical personnel

      (5) Teaches personal responsibility

      (6) Charismatic leader

      (7) Total support

   e. <u>"28 day" programs</u>. Focus on detoxification, support of abstinence, involvement of the whole "family" system, long term outpatient follow-up, usually associated with AA in some manner.

4. **Chemical blockade**

   a. Antabuse for alcoholic:

   (1) Blocks the degradation of acetaldehyde therefore if the alcoholic drinks while taking antabuse, they will develop acetaldehyde poisoning (flushing, nausea and vomiting, tremor, stomach cramps, malaise).

   (2) This is a classical conditioning paradigm where the intent is to establish a learned aversive physiologic reaction to drinking alcohol or even thinking about drinking.

   b. Methadone for narcotics addicts

   (1) Methadone is only useful in treating opioid addiction. To use Methadone, the addict must be associated with a Drug Enforcement Administration (DEA), and State licensed program. There are two types of licenses: Analgesia & Detoxification; and Maintenance.

   (2) Person who may be placed on Methadone Maintenance must be 18 years of age, have a documented two year history of narcotic addiction, and be voluntary.

   (3) Methadone Maintenance programs are rigidly controlled regarding dose level and how many take-home doses the individual may have.

   (4) Maintenance programs are oriented toward substituting methadone for the illicit opiate, until the individual can structure intra- and inter-personal life to not be dependent on chemicals to function. The aim is always to withdraw the persons from the chemical over time.

   (5) The withdrawal syndrome from Methadone is similar to that of other opiates. It is slower in onset and lasts longer.

   (6) Methadone advantages:

   (a) 1 dose lasts 24-36 hours.

   (b) It's a legal drug.

   (c) Blocks narcotic hunger.

    (d)   It is pure, therefore decreased medical complications.

    (e)   No tolerance develops if used as prescribed (oral administration).

    (f)   Delivered in a total rehabilitation package.

    (g)   Inexpensive.

(7)   High success rate on long-term (7-year) follow-up.

    (a)   Increased personal, family, and social responsibility.

    (b)   Methadone clinics have reduced crime rate up to 64%.

CHAPTER 6

THOUGHT DISORDERS

I. PSYCHOSES

A. <u>In general</u>: <u>The term Psychosis is a statement of severity, not a diagnostic entity.</u>

   1. Definition: Disorders which <u>must</u> reach psychotic levels at some time during their course (patients are non-psychotic most of the time).

   Impaired Mental Functioning:

   a. <u>Interfere grossly with the capacity to meet ordinary demands of life; e.g., provide one's own shelter. That is they have very impaired ability to function.</u>

   b. Have grossly impaired sense of reality, reality testing, and adaptation to reality. The term <u>reality testing</u> means "can the person check out internal experience (perception) to find if it is "real or not?"

   c. Results in gross personality disorganization; <u>the person appears bizarre</u>. Speech and behavior is often bizarre and delusions and hallucinations are common. Thoughts are incomprehensible to others and appear illogical.

   d. Grossly <u>disrupt interpersonal (object) relations</u>.

   e. <u>Gross disturbances in memory, perception, and language: (if these are present, probably dealing with an organically based psychosis, not a functional one; see Chapter 4).</u>

   f. <u>Emotions</u>

      (1) Labile

      (2) Flat or blunted

      (3) Inappropriate to content of thought: e.g., laughing about a tragic incident they are describing.

   g. <u>Sense of self</u>

      (1) Loss of ego boundaries

      (2) Severe identity crisis; existential crisis

h. <u>Volition</u>

    (1)   Decreased drive, ambition

    (2)   Ambivalence: can't decide what to do

i. <u>Relationship to external world</u>

    (1)   Withdrawal; detachment

    (2)   Autistic thinking

j. <u>Psychomotor behavior</u>

    (1)   Grimacing, other mannerisms

    (2)   Ritualistic behavior

    (3)   Excessive and inappropriate silliness, aggressiveness, sexuality

    (4)   Catatonic stupor, excitement, rigidity, negativism, posturing

k. <u>Physical symptoms</u>

    (1)   Nonlocalizing neurological "soft" signs

    (2)   Ocular abnormalities

    (3)   Impaired smooth pursuit eye movement

l. <u>All of the above occurs in clear sensorium</u>

2. **Three major types:** Thought Disorders, Affective Disorders (Chapter 7) and some Organic Brain Disorders/Syndromes covered in Chapter 4.

II. THOUGHT DISORDERS

A. Thought disorder is diagnosed in terms of a disruption in the <u>process</u> of thought or the <u>content</u> of thought **in the presence of a clear level of consciousness.**

1. **Process:** too much or too little of:

a. <u>Productivity</u>: flight of ideas; fragmentation; spontaneity; mutism; blocking of thoughts; **echolalia**- echoing what is heard.

b. <u>Continuity</u>: circumstantiality; tangential; intrusive thinking.

c. <u>Additional forms of abnormality</u>: **over-inclusion** (the person's thoughts simply will not come to any logical conclusion); **neologisms** (made up words which have no meaning); **looseness of association**-words put together in sentences that are meaningless, e.g., **"word salad"** or "clanging" where the association is made on the basis of words that sound alike.

2. **Content**

   a. <u>Autistic</u> (has meaning only to the individual) versus logical.

   b. <u>Concrete</u> versus abstract.

   c. <u>Delusional</u>: a false fixed belief system which is not shared by the majority of peers; and not changeable by logic.

   May be: bizarre and confused; persecutory; grandiose; of influence (being controlled by external forces, thought broadcasting [thoughts get out of the head and are audible to others], thought insertion [others put thoughts into the head], thought withdrawal [thoughts are plucked out of the mind]).

   d. <u>Poverty of ideas</u>

3. **Perceptual Disturbances**

   a. <u>Illusions</u>: a misinterpreted sensory experience; e.g., a blowing drape in the shadows is perceived as someone crawling through the window.

   b. <u>Hallucinations</u>: a sensory experience for which there is not adequate external sensory stimulation. Excludes dreams and "after effect". Usually are auditory (voices); but, can be visual, olfactory, tactile, gustatory.

   c. <u>Depersonalization, derealization</u>

   d. <u>Hypersensitivity to sound/sight/smell</u>

B. There are seven subtypes of thought disorders

   1. **Schizophrenia**

      a. <u>In general</u>:

         (1)   A <u>clinical</u> syndrome, not a discrete disease.

         (2)   The most common psychotic disorder.

         (3)   A <u>major</u> public health problem.

         (4)   Usual onset in adolescence or late adolescence.

         (5)   <u>1%</u> of the population is schizophrenic. <u>25%</u> of all new hospital admissions are for schizophrenia. <u>50%</u> of all residents of state institutions are schizophrenics. <u>Many homeless are schizophrenic and constitute a large health care problem.</u>

      b. <u>Etiology</u>: Schizophrenia is best regarded as a group of disorders with multiple interacting causes with expression in a final common pathway.

         (1)   Heredity or Genetics:

             (a)   Possible polygenic mode of inheritance

             (b)   Lifetime risk

- monozygotic twin	40-50%
- dizygotic twins	14%
- sibling of patient	10%

REMEMBER: Monozygotic > Dizygotic > Sibs

- parent of patient	5%
- one parent with disorder	10-15%
- two parents with disorder	30-40%
- general population	1%

         (2)   Anatomical Sites: dysfunctions in the septum, temporal lobes, limbic system and reticular activating system have been implicated.

             (a)   CT scans have demonstrated both enlargement of the lateral and third ventricles and cortical atrophy in a large percent of schizophrenic patients. Some recent studies have suggested that almost all

Schizophrenics have enlarged ventricles relative to control groups (includes sibling controls).

(b) MRI results strongly suggest temporal lobe loss of neurons.

(c) Some PET research has suggested a decrease of blood flow and glucose metabolization in the frontal lobes.

(d) Autopsy findings: Too many D_2 receptors may be present in the basal ganglion and limbic system which would lead to excessive central DA activity.

(e) Some postmortem studies suggest degeneration of various portions of the basal ganglion and limbic system.

(3) Biochemistry:

(a) Most important at this time is the Catecholamine or Dopamine Theory of schizophrenia. This may be due to hyperactive post-synaptic DA receptors.

(b) Norepinephrine is also implicated in Schizophrenia.

(c) Low GABA levels (resulting in disinhibition) also is hypothesized to be involved.

(4) Familial Factors: Core conflict is Trust/Mistrust. Cause-effect is not clear. These are correlations.

(a) Important as precipitants of initial onset as well as relapse; doesn't cause schizophrenia.

(b) Double Bind Hypothesis (Bateson): two conflicting messages are sent to the person, each demanding a response. The victim is not allowed to comment on the bind and may not leave the field. E.g., a parent says to a child, "Don't do everything I tell you to do." While this theory has some validity, one finds these communications in other families.

(c) Parenting: (Jacque Schiff): dysfunctional parents transmit three statements to the child:

1) Parents come first.
2) You are no good.
3) Outside world is dangerous.

(d) Often find extreme "emotional closeness" and very high expression of emotions particularly hostility.

(e) "Schizophrenogenic" mothers. Early it was observed that the mothers of schizophrenics were "cold" and often were referred to as "ice-box mothers". This was initially thought to be etiologic; however, it has subsequently been established that this was a reaction to the schizophrenic child, not the cause of the schizophrenia.

(5) Socio-cultural

(a) Apparently schizophrenia occurs in all cultures

(b) Predominance in lower SES classes and slum areas of cities. May reflect persons who cannot adequately care for themselves or compete, drifting to slums where demands for performance are less; and public support systems (e.g., "missions") are present. Low SES environments don't cause the disease; however, they do render it difficult to treat.

(c) There has been observed a higher rate of schizophrenia among first generation immigrants. It is assumed that this is secondary to the stress of relocation in persons who are predisposed to the disease.

c. The DSM-III-R diagnostic criteria for schizophrenia include:

(1) Symptoms must last at least 6 months.

(2) There is a deterioration from the previous characteristic level of occupational, interpersonal, and self-supportive functioning.

(3) <u>Actively psychotic</u> during at least part of the 6 months (at least one week)

(4) Delusions: incoherence or marked **loosening of associations; catatonic behavior; flat or grossly inappropriate affect; bizarre delusions.**

(5) Prominent hallucinations: running commentary, or 2 or more voices conversing with each other for extended periods of time.

d. The concept of positive symptoms and negative symptoms is often useful clinically.

(1) Positive symptoms are active in nature and give the person with Schizophrenia an unusual, often bizarre appearance. They include:

  (a) Strange behaviors: public sexual behavior, marked agitation accompanied by aggressiveness, odd dress, etc..

  (b) A clear thought disorder: illogical, looseness of association, circumstantial, tangential, clang associations, word salad, etc.

  (c) Hallucinations: in any sensory modality. Auditory are often organized conversations.

  (d) Delusions: belief that people are inserting or withdrawing thoughts from their head; persecutory, grandiose, religious, somatic, etc..

(2) Negative symptoms give the person the appearance of inactivity, dullness, and retardation. They include:

  (a) Absence, poverty or slowness of speech.

  (b) Flat affect and emotional unresponsiveness. Speech has no melody.

  (c) Impaired volition, poor grooming and hygiene, little energy.

  (d) Anhedonia in recreation, sexual activity, socialization.

  (e) Poor attention in social situations.

e. <u>Course</u>: most common course is one of acute exacerbations with increasing residual impairment between episodes.

(1)   Prodromal phase

(a)   Deterioration of functioning

(b)   Symptoms develop variably

(c)   "Prepsychotic personality" (Socially inept; poor school performance in spite of adequate intelligence; shy and socially withdrawn).

(2)   Active phase

(a)   Psychotic symptoms prominent

(b)   May be stress precipitated

(c)   Usually in late teens or early 20's

(3)   Residual phase

(a)   Similar to prodromal but more dysfunctional and mildly psychotic

(b)   Most of life spent here (i.e. not in active phase)

(4)   General comments

(a)   25% need sheltered living or chronic inpatient care.

(b)   Gradual deteriorating course over time.

f. <u>Sub-Types of Schizophrenia</u>

In general: overlapping symptoms; shifting diagnoses; paranoid vs non-paranoid is a major distinction; final common picture of custodial care.

(1)   **Schizophrenia, Disorganized Type**

No <u>systematized</u> delusions

<u>Incoherence, marked loosening of associations, grossly disorganized behavior</u>

<u>Flat, blunted or grossly inappropriate affect (e.g. strikingly silly)</u>.

(2) **Schizophrenia, Catatonic Type:** Major striking feature is <u>disturbed motor activity</u> (either extremely agitated or extremely stuporous to the point of no movement whatsoever.)

Especially marked with catatonic schizophrenia is "waxy flexibility" (place their extremities in a position, and they will hold that position for a protracted period of time.) There may also be stupor or mutism, negativism, rigidity, voluntary posturing, or excitement (purposeless and not influenced by external stimuli).

(3) **Schizophrenia, Paranoid Type:** Major feature is <u>disturbed thoughts</u>. Has systematized delusions usually of persecution/ grandeur or jealousy. Develops later than other types and stable over time. May be aggressive, angry or fearful. May have auditory hallucinations of a single theme.

They rarely demonstrate incoherence, marked loose associations, flat or grossly inappropriate affect, catatonic behavior, or grossly disorganized behavior

<u>The most stable and the best prognosis of the different subtypes.</u>

(4) **Schizophrenia, Undifferentiated Type:** Display the signs and symptoms of schizophrenia; however, there is no one group of prominent symptoms present long enough to allow classification above.

(5) **Schizophrenia, Residual Type:** History of a previous schizophrenic episode; however, at present does not display major symptoms. In partial remission. May have minor signs of less severe symptoms (e.g. social isolation and withdrawal; impairment in role function; peculiar behavior; impaired hygiene; odd beliefs; lack of interest/initiative; etc.).

g. <u>Treatment</u>: must be tailored to the individual patient and their life situation.

(1) Antipsychotic medications are almost universally used in these patients. All antipsychotics have shown effectiveness over placebos in double blind studies.

(2) Patients are only placed in secured psychiatric hospitals during times of exacerbations of the most florid and disruptive symptoms.

(3) Rehabilitation/resocialization/re-education is a major total thrust for the care and treatment of these patients. Sheltered living facilities, sheltered workshops, day hospitals and day treatment centers are all used interchangeably to maintain the patient at the most independent and functional level.

(4) Behavior modification: reward systems (e.g., Token Economy) to shape social behavior.

(5) Group therapy/group process to promote support and socialization.

(6) Family intervention/therapy/support to prevent stress on the patient and consequent exacerbation of the disease.

(7) Psychotherapy: individual psychotherapy (supportive & reality oriented).

h. Prognosis

(1) General considerations

   (a) Variable levels of dysfunction: some are not as disturbed as others, and some have a minimal number of symptoms and episodes.

   (b) Legal problems: if there are legal problems (usually as a result of the positive symptoms), the stress of the interface with the legal system may attenuate the prognosis.

   (c) Increased mortality particularly in those who are "homeless" and have minimal health care available; remember these persons have difficulty taking care of themselves; suicide rate is 10%.

(2) Drug treatment has reduced the length of hospitalization and the quantity of suffering; but, the long term (twenty year) follow up has not changed.

(3)   In favor of better prognosis:

    (a)   Late onset: onset after age 30.

    (b)   Well socialized premorbid behavior: good premorbid personality development and functioning.

    (c)   No familial history of schizophrenia.

    (d)   Marked confusion and affect during acute episode.

    (e)   A precipitating stress.

    (f)   Acute onset.

    (g)   Family history of Mood Disorder.

    (h)   Normal CT scan.

2. **Brief reactive psychosis:**

a. Acute psychotic episode of <u>up to one month duration</u> after a severe emotional stress event.

b. <u>Symptoms</u>: extreme agitation and turmoil in behavior with gross deterioration of personality (Positive symptoms).

c. More common in some personality disorders, but generally no pre-morbid suggestion of "break down".

d. <u>Treatment</u>

    (1)   Medications if the patient is agitated or highly emotional.

    (2)   Hospitalization if the patient's safety is compromised by the condition.

    (3)   Psychotherapy to manage the stressor event.

e. Recovery is quick and complete if the stress is well managed.

3. **Schizophreniform Disorder:**

a. Differentiated from schizophrenia and brief reactive psychosis by time. Is <u>more than two weeks but less than six months</u>.

b. Form is similar to schizophrenia except more acute onset and agitation; and more sudden resolution.

c. Persons usually had better premorbid adjustment and better post-recovery functioning.

d. Some mild increased prevalence of schizophrenia in the family.

e. Often go on to develop schizophrenia.

f. Treatment: like that for the acute schizophrenic episode.

4. **Schizo-Affective Disorder:** Both schizophrenia and major affective disorder elements are present.

a. Inadequately documented disorder. Is probably not a true separate diagnostic entity. Diagnosis of exclusion.

b. Evidence of both Schizophrenia and Major Mood Disorder (Bipolar or Major Depressive Disorder) concurrently.

c. Relatives have higher rates of either Schizophrenia or mood disorders.

d. Treatment: Depends upon the symptoms being manifested by the patient.

   (1)   Concurrent use of antipsychotics and medications for affective disorders is indicated.

   (2)   There is some indication that ECT is useful when medications are not effective.

e. Between Schizophrenia and Bipolar Disorder in prognosis.

5. **Delusional (Paranoid) Disorder (Paranoia):**

a. Do NOT have flat or inappropriate affect, hallucinations, or markedly bizarre delusions.

b. DO have one or more delusions of grandiosity, jealousy, persecution or somatic illness; which are specific and well organized (encapsulated).

c. Later in onset, often associated with immigration or emigration (Migration Psychosis), or other severe stress.

d. No pervasive disturbances of mood and thought.

e. Seem normal until delusional system recognized.

f. May be hypersensitive, mistrustful, litigious.

g. Social isolates with good occupational functioning.

h. Must last at least one month.

i. Treatment:

    (1) Medications for symptoms, e.g., anxiety. Antipsychotics aren't generally helpful.

    (2) Individual psychotherapy.

6. **Induced Psychotic Disorder (Shared Paranoid Disorder):**

a. Delusion develops which is shared with another person. First person usually had a previous psychotic disorder diagnosis, and the second was not psychotic prior to the onset of the induced delusion. Sometimes referred to as a "folie a deux."

b. Delusional system develops in a second person as a result of a close relationship with the first person who has a psychotic disorder with prominent delusions.

c. Delusions: share content - often believable.

d. First (psychotic) person usually dominant over passive (and initially healthy) second person.

e. Socially isolated.

f. Quite rare, therefore little is known about etiology or treatment.

g. Treatment:

    (1) Separation usually helps the second person.

    (2) Treat the first person for their psychotic condition.

7. **Psychotic Disorder Not Otherwise Specified (Atypical Psychosis):** Most common use of this classification is when there is insufficient information to make a diagnosis or the psychotic level symptoms don't fit another diagnostic group.

CHAPTER 7

MOOD DISORDERS

I.   **NORMAL MOOD STATES**

   A. <u>Sadness</u>: It is universal and a part of life. The normal
      response to the experience of loss of a significant object
      (person).

   B. <u>Grief</u> (Uncomplicated Bereavement)

      1. More profound; greater stress

      2. May go to full depressive syndrome

   C. <u>Simply feeling sad doesn't constitute depression</u>; and grief
      reaction should not be misdiagnosed as depression.

II. **DISORDERS OF MOOD**

   A. <u>Definition of Depression</u>: A group of disorders whose
      common and essential feature is a disturbance of mood
      accompanied by related cognitive, psychomotor,
      psychophysiological, and interpersonal problems.

      1. **Mood or emotional symptoms**

         a. Depressed mood

         b. Irritability

         c. Anhedonia (loss of interest)

         d. Social withdrawal

         e. Preoccupation with death

         f. Sad faces, tearful

      2. **Cognitive**

         a. Guilt, worthlessness, self-criticism

         b. Despair, hopelessness

         c. Distractible, impaired concentration

         d. Indecisive, uncertain

         e. Obsessional, hypochondriacal

f. Impaired memory

g. Delusions, hallucinations

3. **Psychomotor and physiologic findings**

   a. Decreased energy, easy fatigability

   b. Insomnia, hypersomnia

   c. Increased or decreased appetite

   d. Increased or decreased weight

   e. Psychomotor agitation or retardation; slow moving, stooped

   f. Decreased libido (sexual or pleasurable interest)

   g. Diurnal variation

   h. Dry mouth, skin

   i. Constipation

4. **The Depressive Syndrome** (can occur in major or minor proportion)

   a. <u>Dysphoria</u> (feeling bad or down) must be present;

   b. <u>AND</u> at least five of the following must be present in the same two-week period:

      (1) Sleep disturbance (too much or too little)

      (2) Appetite and weight change

      (3) Decreased enjoyment/sex (**anhedonia**).

      (4) Feelings of guilt, self reproach, worthlessness

      (5) Suicidal ideas/plans/actions; recurrent thoughts of death. <u>**Suicide is a serious danger in depression**</u>.

      (6) Agitation/retardation of movements

      (7) Decreased concentration

      (8) Decreased energy/easy fatigue

c. <u>In adolescents</u>, the signs and symptoms of depression include withdrawal, decreased school performance, substance abuse, delinquency, and promiscuity.

d. <u>Depressive Syndrome appears in physical illnesses</u>, sometimes as the presenting complaint: post partum, post myocardial infarction (where it leads to poor compliance), liver disease, lung cancer, pancreatitis, alcoholism, AIDS, etc..

e. <u>Depressive illness is the most overlooked mental disorder in America.</u>

B. <u>Definition of Mania</u>: There must be positive symptoms present. These include the following.

1. **Manic Symptoms**

   a. <u>Emotional</u>

      (1)   Euphoria, excited

      (2)   Emotional lability

      (3)   Irritability

      (4)   Egocentric, demanding, low frustration tolerance

   b. <u>Cognitive</u>

      (1)   Elevated self esteem

      (2)   Speech disturbances

            - Loud, intrusive
            - Rhyming (clang associations)
            - Pressured
            - Flight of ideas
            - Incoherent

      (3)   Impaired judgement

      (4)   Persecutory and grandiose ideation

      (5)   Delusions, hallucinations

       c. <u>Physiologic</u>

          (1)   Increased energy

          (2)   Insomnia, decreased need for sleep

          (3)   Decreased appetite

   2. **Manic syndrome**

       a. <u>Euphoria</u>: A period of abnormally and persistently elevated, expansive, or irritable mood.

       b. <u>Three of the following</u>:

          (1)   Inflated self esteem (can be delusional grandiosity)

          (2)   Decreased need for sleep

          (3)   Pressure to talk

          (4)   Racing thoughts or flight of ideas

          (5)   Distractibility (impaired attention)

          (6)   Increased goal-directed activity (social, occupational, sexual) or physical restlessness; agitation; excitability.

          (7)   Excessive involvement in pleasurable activities that have high potential for painful consequences, e.g., buying sprees, excessive sexual behavior, foolish business investments.

III.   ETIOLOGY OF MOOD DISORDERS:

A. <u>Heredity possibilities</u>.

B. May represent a type of <u>biological rhythm</u>.

C. In psychosocial theory, it is assumed that particularly the depressive aspects are reactions to loss, while other people feel that the depression may be a technique to "blackmail" others into "caring for the patient."

D. In psychodynamic theory depression is often seen as anger, which should rightfully be placed on someone else. However, the angry person deems the anger to be inappropriate and turns the anger in on the self to punish the self for being angry with the other person.

Often one finds the loss of a significant other early in the life of the indicated patient. E.g., a father died or deserted the family and was not replaced by a "surrogate father."

E. "Learned Helplessness": The individual has a series of defeating experiences in their life. No matter how hard they have tried they couldn't overcome the defeating object or condition. They then "give up" and quit trying, even though later the defeating object or condition is no longer present.

F. Cognitive model: <u>Automatic</u> negative thoughts have learned to be associated to given situations, persons, behaviors. These negative thoughts or cognitions lead to negative feelings, which over time become chronic in nature and result in depressed affect as the characteristic condition of the person.

G. There is a catecholamine hypothesis involving norepinephrine. E.g., too little norepinephrine results in depressed affect; and too much results in mania.

At this time, mood disorders are recognized to be much more complex in biochemical substrates than one neurotransmitter system.

IV. **CLASSIFICATION (SYNDROMES):** Must have interfered with work, social life, or become dangerous to self or others.

Clinical Mood Disorders

Psychotic
- <u>Bipolar Disorder</u>
- <u>Major Depressive Disorder</u>

Nonpsychotic
- <u>Cyclothymia</u>
- <u>Dysthymia</u>

V. **PSYCHOTIC LEVEL MOOD DISORDERS:** Bipolar Disorder and Major Depressive Disorder.

    A. <u>Bipolar Disorder</u> (Depressed, Mixed, Manic)

        1. **Predisposition**

            a. <u>Genetic factors</u>

                (1)   15% prevalence in first degree relatives for an affective disorder

                (2)   Polygenic inheritance

            b. Has 1% lifetime risk

            c. Male to female ratio is equal.

        2. **Background Information**

            a. Note that mania at some time, severe enough to produce impaired functioning, **is necessary** to establish this diagnosis.

            b. 80 - 90% have depressive episodes

            c. Can be psychotic (20% have delusions and/or hallucinations)

            d. Cyclic course varies

        3. **Course of the illness**

            a. First episode late adolescence or early adulthood, often manic (in 60-80% of cases). Age of onset is 30-35 years.

            b. Onset sudden, mania lasts approximately 4 months if not treated, and depression for approximately one year

            c. Course is chronic with majority depressive episodes and increasing frequency during first 10 years, then fewer episodes (average 7-9 over lifetime).

            d. Suicide, legal/financial problems, drug abuse are major problems

        4. **Characterized by:**

            a. No obvious precipitating factor (i.e., endogenous);

b. Psychomotor changes;

c. Usually a number of episodes and <u>full recovery between attacks</u>.

5. **Illness is more frequent in upper SES classes than in lower. One of the exceptions to low SES being correlated with severe mental illness.**

6. **Subtypes**

   a. <u>Bipolar Disorder, Depressed Type</u>: Has had one or more manic episodes and is currently in a depressive episode.

   b. <u>Bipolar Disorder, Mixed Type</u>:

   Currently displaying both manic and depressive episodes either intermixed or alternating every few days.

   c. <u>Bipolar Disorder, Manic Type</u>:

   Currently in a manic episode.

7. **Treatment**

   a. <u>Anti-manics</u>: The major breakthrough in treatment of bipolar illness has been lithium salts. If patient is unresponsive to lithium, carbamazepine (Tegretol) is often useful.

   b. If patient is very agitated when first seen, often antipsychotics are indicated to reduce the agitation; and are discontinued when the agitated behavior is no longer present.

   c. Psychotherapy to deal with the sequelae of the disorder: e.g., legal involvement, environmental triggers, marital dysfunction, concomitant substance abuse, etc..

B. <u>Major Depressive Disorder</u>

  1. **Background data:**

   a. <u>Predisposition</u>

    (1) Higher social strata

    (2)   Genetic correlates seen in relatives

        - Major Depression
        - Alcoholism
        - Antisocial Personality Disorder

      (a)   First-degree relatives have 17% prevalence

    (3)   Alcoholism

    (4)   Chronic stress

    (5)   Being female

b. <u>Lifetime prevalence</u>: males=2-4%; females=5-9% (e.g., M:F=1:2).

c. Precipitating event found in almost 25% (50% in the elderly).

d. Sometimes accompanied by a thought disorder.

e. Onset at any age but usually in adulthood where it is spread throughout the ages.

f. 85% have more than one episode.

2. **Course**

a. More severe signs and symptoms of depression

b. Diurnal variation/Seasonal variation

c. <u>Clinical course</u>:

    (1)   Begins over 1-3 weeks; lasts 3-8 months if not treated; disabled during episode

    (2)   40% full recovery

    (3)   40% episodic

    (4)   20% chronic

    (5)   One in five patients will stay depressed through two years even with treatment. Only 15% will never have another episode.

    (6)   15% commit suicide (30X the rate of the general population)

3. **Diagnosis:** Presence of depressive syndrome with many of the more serious symptoms. Has never had a manic episode. Are profoundly depressed. See a profound metabolic shutdown/slowdown.

   a. <u>Other Subtypes</u>

      (1) Melancholia: Vegetative symptoms: anhedonic, severe insomnia, worse in the morning, psychomotor changes, and anorexia with weight loss.

         Responds well to medications and ECT.

      (2) Post-partum depression: Following the birth of a child.

      (3) Seasonal affective disorder (SAD): Occurs at the same time of year (usually winter) for at least 3 years. Absent during other times of the year.

      (4) Double depression: may have more than one type of diagnosable depressive illness: e.g., Major Depressive Disorder and Dysthymia.

      (5) Masked depression: Depression which is manifested in the patient by another condition. The most common of these are:

         (a) Substance abuse

         (b) Acting-out behavior: e.g., hypersexuality, stealing, etc.

         (c) Anxiety: presenting symptoms are those of generalized anxiety, with diffuse feelings of "impending doom".

         (d) Somatic complaints (headache, GI distress, etc.)

         (e) Chronic Fatigue.

         (f) Insomnia

4. **Depression can be assessed with the following instruments:**

   a. Beck Depression Inventory,

   b. Zung Self-Rating Depression Scale,

   c. Hamilton Depression Rating Scale.

5. **Treatment**

   a. <u>Medications</u>:

      (1)   Heterocyclic or newer antidepressants

      (2)   MAO inhibitors for non-responders to the heterocyclics

      (3)   Antipsychotics if the person is psychotically depressed.

      (4)   Anxiolytics for associated anxiety symptoms

   b. <u>Psychotherapy</u> to work through the loss/grief mourning reaction, or the anger.

      (1)   Supportive: to help the person through crisis precipitating situations.

      (2)   Behavioral: to improve the persons level of active functioning. E.g., to get out of bed, resocialize, etc..

      (3)   Cognitive: to change automatic negative cognitions.

      (4)   Psychoanalytically oriented: to deal with early losses and their sequelae

      (5)   Family/Couples/Group: to work through situations that are contributory to the depressed affect; and, to decrease the impact of the affective disorder on the family unit.

   c. <u>Electro-Convulsive Therapy (ECT)</u> is a viable alternative particularly in some psychotic level mood disorders, e.g., Major Depressive Disorder with Melancholia.

VI. **NON-PSYCHOTIC (MINOR) MOOD DISORDERS**

A. <u>Dysthymia (Depressive Neurosis)</u>: Defined as a non-psychotic disorder of lowered mood and/or anhedonia (lack of pleasure) for at least two years and never with a two-month period free of symptoms. This is a common disorder.

1. **Predisposition**

    a. <u>Major childhood loss</u>: a major parenting figure is lost in the first few years of life and is not replaced;

    b. <u>Chronic stress</u>;

    c. Psychiatric conditions, pre-existing or co-existing;

    d. <u>Being female</u>: it is more common in women (3-4:1).

2. Feel depressed, have difficulty falling asleep, <u>feel best in the morning</u>, and despondent in the afternoon and evening. Can display any of the non-psychotic signs and symptoms of depression.

    Mild, non-psychotic signs and symptoms of depression, less severe than Major Depression.

3. Often develops for the first time in childhood, adolescence or early adulthood. Usually begins late 20's or 30's.

4. Exacerbated by the loss of a person, health, job, or by chronic stress such as a medical disorder.

5. Insidious onset, chronic course - must be symptomatic for at least two years.

6. Treatment: usually psychotherapy is the indicated intervention modality.

B. <u>Cyclothymia</u>:

1. Presence of mild depression <u>and</u> hypomania (less than manic level) either separately or mixed continuously or intermittently over at least a two year period. No two month period free of symptoms.

2. Begins in adolescence to early 20's.

3. More common in women (2:1).

4. Chronically disabling pattern which yields troubled interpersonal relationships, job instability, occasionally suicide attempts and short hospitalization. Marked drug and alcohol abuse.

5. Predisposition - family history of Major Mood Disorder (esp. Bipolar disorder); being female.

6. Sub-clinical Bipolar Disorder - 35% develop a major mood disorder.

7. **Treatment**

   a. <u>Medications</u>: Lithium is indicated.

   b. Psychotherapy to stabilize life and relationships. Also family/couples/marital to deal with the impact of the disorder on the life of the person.

CHAPTER 8

"NEUROSES"

I. GENERAL INTRODUCTION

A. The next three sections (Anxiety Disorders, Dissociative Disorders, and Somatoform Disorders) earlier were called "neuroses"; however, <u>that term is no longer used</u> in the classification of Mental Disorders.

B. These are disorders characterized by underlying anxiety either directly experienced or controlled automatically by defense mechanisms.

  1. Therefore the disorder is experienced as uncomfortable <u>symptoms</u> which the patient feels are foolish and fights against. <u>They are ego dystonic</u>.

  2. Usually abrupt development; usually in adulthood.

  3. No gross misinterpretation of reality or personality disorganization, i.e., they are not psychotic.

  4. While most appear to be learned, recent research is suggesting a more biologic etiology for some.

C. There are two concepts which are important in these conditions.

  1. **Primary gain:** what the symptom does for the patient's internal psychic economy, e.g., prevents overwhelming of the ego.

  2. **Secondary gain:** what the symptom gets the patient, e.g., sympathy, attention, avoidance of responsibility.

II. THE DIAGNOSTIC GROUPS

A. <u>Group One: The Anxiety Disorders</u>

<u>IMPORTANT</u>: must differentiate anxiety states from hypoxia, stimulant toxicity, hyperthyroidism, etc..

For this group of disorders, a number of medications of the anxiolytic and antidepressant type are very useful.

  1. **Phobic Disorders:**

    a. Intense fear of an object or situation.

    b. Usually the object or situation of which the person is fearful is <u>not</u> the true feared object. The object feared is being <u>displaced</u> upon.

    c. Encounter with the object or situation produces fear.

    d. Person avoids phobic object or situation.

    e. Recognizes the fear is excessive or unreasonable.

    f. The person fears he will experience humiliation or embarrassment.

    g. <u>Treatment</u>: Medications and behavior modification to desensitize the person to the feared object.

2. **Panic Disorder (without Agoraphobia):**

    a. Has dramatic, acute symptoms lasting minutes to hours, is self limiting, and occurs in patients with or without chronic anxiety.

    b. The symptoms are perceived by the patient and those around him as medical and are characteristic of strong autonomic discharge (heart pounding, chest pain, trembling, choking, abdominal pain, sweating, dizziness, as well as disorganization, confusion, dread, and occasionally a sense of impending doom or terror).

    c. In the early stage of the disorder, may have multiple episodes which last for variable lengths of time. Later in the course of the illness, if appropriately treated the episodes may occur very briefly (a few seconds) on an infrequent basis.

    d. A typical panic attack can be produced by the intravenous infusion of sodium lactate in patients with panic disorder but not in normals.

    e. Most also develop **Agoraphobia** (fear of being in places from which escape might be difficult). This has a higher prevalence in women. Note: Agoraphobia can occur without panic disorder.

        (1) The patient reports that he is fearful of embarrassing self in public.

    f. Disruption of important interpersonal relations may be a precursor of panic disorders.

    g. Runs in families and occurs equally in men and women. Some had childhood episode of separation anxiety.

    h. <u>Treatment</u>: Antidepressant medication, anxiolytics and individual therapy (behavior modification, supportive types).

3. **Generalized Anxiety Disorder:**

   a. Anxiety is subjectively experienced and accompanied by:

      (1)   Motor symptoms of tension, e.g. tremor, restlessness

      (2)   Autonomic hyperactivity; dyspnea, palpitations, sweating/cold clammy hands, dry mouth, dizziness, gastrointestinal distress, polyuria.

      (3)   Vigilance and scanning: "on edge," restless, exaggerated startle response, concentration problems, sleep problems, irritable.

   b. **Symptoms must last six months** during which there may be a few symptom free days.

   c. The core issue in this disorder is the patient does not have awareness of what is triggering the anxious condition.

   d. <u>Treatment</u> is anti-anxiety medications and psychotherapy to isolate and deal with the dynamic etiologic event in the patient's background.

4. **Obsessive-Compulsive Disorder:**

   a. Obsessions: thoughts, (e.g., contamination, aggression, sexual, somatic, need for symmetry) about things and people. E.g., obsessive thoughts might be fear of killing one's child.

   b. Compulsions: behaviors, e.g., checking, cleaning, counting things. Compulsive urges may be urges to clean the dryer with an astringent between drying loads of clothes.

   c. Core conflict is <u>control</u>, usually control of time, dirt and/or money.

   d. More common in females than in males.

   e. <u>Treatment</u>: medications; especially serotonergic antidepressants; dynamic psychotherapy to deal with the control issues; and behavior modification to modulate the compulsive behaviors.

      Stereotactic psychosurgery is under investigation at this time.

5. **Post-traumatic Stress Disorder:**

   a. There must be the existence of a recognizable stressor that would evoke significant symptoms of stress in almost anyone (e.g. war, rape, etc.).

   b. The symptoms include re-experiencing trauma through recollection of the trauma in the awake state or in dreams. Can also be recollected as sudden feelings as if the traumatic event was reoccurring.

   c. Numbing of responsiveness and reduced involvement with the external world.

   d. Persons with the disorder have at least two of the following that were not present before the trauma: hyper-alertness, exaggerated startle response or sleep disturbance, guilt about surviving where others have not, memory impairment/trouble concentrating, avoiding activities which arouse recollection of the traumatic event, and intensification of symptoms by exposure to events which symbolize or resemble the traumatic event.

   e. Resentment is a common element in PTSD patients.

   f. Many of these patients also show concomitant problems with:

      (1)   Chemical abuse

      (2)   Aggression-violence: particularly when re-experiencing the traumatic episode or something similar to it.

   g. Two subtypes:

      (1)   **Acute**, where the symptoms occur within six months of the trauma;

      (2)   **Chronic or delayed**, where onset of symptoms appears six months after the trauma; and/or the symptoms persist for months to decades.

   h. NOTE: some researchers think there is a biologic predisposition which is triggered by environmental events.

   i. Treatment:

      (1)   Antidepressant medications have been useful in some persons. Antianxiety preparations should be used sparingly because of the abuse potential.

    (2)   Group therapy, where catharsis of the conflict is encouraged and the person is supported, has been very helpful.

    (3)   Expression of resentment for the stressing event is central to resolution of the conflict.

B. <u>Group Two:</u> <u>Dissociative Disorders</u> (no known biologic etiology)

1. **Psychogenic Amnesia:**

   a. Sudden inability to recall important personal information. Too extensive to be explained by ordinary forgetfulness. Usually begins after severe stress. E.g., a woman blocking out the memory of the face of the man who raped her.

   b. Treatment: Psychotherapy to resolve conflicted issue.

2. **Psychogenic Fugue:**

   a. Sudden unexpected travel away from home or one's place of work with inability to recall one's past. Frequent assumption of a new identity, either partial or complete.

   b. The classic situation where the man goes for a package of cigarettes and never comes back.

   c. Usually lasts a few hours or days, but may continue for months. Usually an abrupt recovery of the memory.

   d. Treatment: Assistance in recovering previous identity. Sometimes includes hypnosis or hypnotic drug assistance.

3. **Multiple Personality:**

   a. The "Three Faces of Eve". Existence within one body of <u>two or more</u> distinct personalities which are dominant at alternate times. The personality that is dominant at a particular time determines individual's behavior. Each personality is complex and integrated with its own unique pattern of social behavior.

   b. Sometimes each has a distinct EEG pattern, eyeglass prescription, etc. When the person moves from one personality into the other, there is usually a brief altered state of consciousness when the patient closes the eyes as the shift in personality is made.

    c. Personalities usually represent poles of behavior (e.g. "a good personality vs. a bad personality"). Sometimes one will have a diagnosable mental disorder and the other will not. Usually the split in the personalities represents the person's inability to integrate positive and negative impulses into one "ego".

    d. Most of these patients show massively dysfunctional parenting in their background; and many have been the victims of severe child abuse (battering, sexual abuse and neglect).

    e. <u>Treatment</u>: psychotherapy to allow the different personalities to integrate into one multifaceted person.

4. Depersonalization Disorder:

    a. Ego-dystonic feelings of unreality or separation from oneself, one's body (depersonalization: e.g., floating to the corner of the room and observing the scene), or one's surroundings (derealization: e.g., suddenly not recognizing where one is).

    b. May report feeling like an automaton.

    c. Differential diagnosis is drug induced states or schizophrenia. Major differential sign is that in this disorder <u>reality testing is intact</u>.

    d. <u>Treatment</u>: Supportive psychotherapy is indicated. Psychopharmacologic intervention has not been successful.

C. <u>Group Three: Somatoform Disorders</u>

1. Somatization Disorder:

    a. History of physical symptoms of several years duration for which no pathophysiology is found, but for which the person has taken medication.

    b. Tend to see many different physicians; and, many patients receive unwarranted surgeries, multiple medications that the physicians are unaware others are prescribing; and, other medical procedures.

    c. Rarely diagnosed in males. Tends to be familial.

d. <u>These patients tend to have a positive review of systems</u>. There must be 13 symptoms from a total list of 35 symptoms in the DSM-III-R. These symptoms fall in the following categories:

(1) Conversion/pseudoneurological: e.g., paralysis.

(2) Gastrointestinal: e.g. nausea and vomiting.

(3) Female reproductive: e.g., painful menstruation.

(4) Psychosexual: e.g., dyspareunia.

(5) Pain: e.g., low back pain.

(6) Cardiopulmonary symptoms: e.g., shortness of breath.

e. <u>Treatment</u>

(1) Psychotherapy to learn to cope with the symptoms.

(2) Medications are contraindicated in most instances.

2. **Conversion Disorder**

a. Disorders of special senses or the voluntary nervous system; e.g. blindness/ motor paralysis. In the motor/sensory symptoms, the distribution of deficit does not follow neuro-anatomic distributions.

b. <u>IMPORTANT</u>: in this disorder, an extensive medical workup is very important since there is research that indicates a significant number of these persons develop true physiologic problems in the relatively near future.

c. Often a lack of concern ("la belle indifference").

d. Rule out malingering, psychophysiologic reactions.

e. Usually the symptom is symbolic of the conflict. For example, if a person does not like their job, they may develop a symptom that does not allow them to work. Note that in psychophysiologic reactions, there is no symbolic expression (conversion defense mechanism). Loss or alteration of function is not intentionally produced.

f. <u>Treatment</u>: Dynamic psychotherapy to establish and work through the conflicts associated with the disorder.

3. **Somatoform Pain Disorder**

a. Preoccupation with pain for at least 6 months in the absence of adequate findings to explain the pain or intensity.

b. The pain is inconsistent with the anatomic distribution of the nervous system. When there is related (underlying) organic pathology, the complaint is in excess of what is expected from physical findings.

c. One can usually establish a temporal relationship between environmental events and exacerbation or initiation of the pain. It allows the individual to avoid some activity and derive environmental support.

d. Depression is a common accompaniment in many of these persons.

e. <u>Treatment</u>

   (1) Behavior modification procedures are helpful in a large percentage of patients.

   (2) Analgesics and antianxiety medications should be avoided. They don't generally help and addiction is a potential complication.

   (3) Antidepressant medications assist some.

4. **Hypochondriasis**

a. Preoccupation with one's body and misinterpretation of physical signs as evidence of presumed disease not supported by physical evaluation.

b. <u>Treatment</u>: medical supportive psychotherapy and education is about the most psychologic care these patients can tolerate.

CHAPTER 9

PERSONALITY DISORDERS

I. GENERAL CONSIDERATIONS

A. <u>Personality</u> refers to a person's relatively stable way of behaving and relating. When these become so intense, rigid, or maladaptive as to cause difficulty between a person and his environment, a personality disorder is said to exist.

B. <u>Personality Disorders are characterized by</u>:

1. **Life long:** recognized in adolescence, but not diagnosed there because most adolescents have behavior that looks like a personality disorder at some time.

2. **It is maladaptive behavior,** not symptoms. Maladaptive behavior in:

   a. relationships

   b. adjustments to society

   c. pursuit of instinctual goals

3. **Usually anxiety is absent** except when there is external stress. Often tolerate stress poorly so minor problems of living lead to anxiety and depression. Premorbid history of seriously ill psychiatric patients often reveals a pre-existing personality disorder.

4. **Ego-syntonic.** Behaviors/symptoms that don't bother self--bother others.

   a. These are interpersonal, not intrapersonal.

   b. It's always someone else's fault. Patients with personality disorders disown personal responsibility for what another feels, attribute blame to others and have difficulty appreciating what they have inflicted on another.

   c. An obvious exception is the dependent personality disorder who takes excessive responsibility for others.

   d. Caveat on this: it does bother self when it isn't working. I.e., if the behavior pattern doesn't work, may become anxious and/or depressed.

5. It is important to be able to differentiate personality
disorders from neurotic or psychotic disorders. Anxiety
and depression are common presenting complaints in each
of these conditions. Basically, individuals with
personality disorders react to stress by attempting to
change the external environment; and secondly, character
deficits are seen as acceptable and part of the self.

6. The importance of recognizing personality disorders in
the practice of medicine is that a number of doctor-
patient difficulties emerge from individuals who have
these chronic, habitual maladaptive modes of proceeding
in this world. These patients:

a. are ambulatory

b. are maladaptive and ultimately come to the attention
of medical personnel

c. have behavioral maladaptation therefore they
ultimately get into difficulty and engage the health
professionals

d. unless managed appropriately will be a mess in any
practice or setting (steal for money, don't keep
appointments, demanding, threatening)

C. Etiology

1. Some research suggests familial factors for some of the
Personality Disorders (Schizotypal, Antisocial and
Borderline).

2. Developmental factors:

a. Adults rewarded maladaptive behavior.

b. Parents of the same sex modeled the behavior.

c. Circumstances prevented developing normal behavior.

3. Characterized by rigid and inappropriate use of one or a
few defense mechanisms.

4. Most are probably learned. Taught through frustration,
models, and experience.

II. DESCRIPTIONS

   A. Cluster A: Individuals seem odd or eccentric.

      1. Paranoid Personality Disorder:

         a. Interprets others' behaviors as deliberately
             demeaning or threatening.

         b. Hypersensitive, suspicious; jealous and envious;
             blaming others.

         c. Quick counterattack, holds grudges.

         d. E.g., the person who takes a joke seriously and
             counters with a vicious attack.

      2. Schizoid Personality Disorder:

         a. Indifferent to social relations.

         b. Shy, reclusive, avoids close relationships;
             daydreaming but no loss of reality testing;
             difficulty in expressing ordinary aggressivity.

         c. No close friends, indifferent to social rewards,
             chooses solitary activity.

         d. E.g., the quiet and strange person in grade school
             and junior high school who disappeared when they
             turned 16.

      3. Schizotypal Personality Disorder:

         a. Have features of schizoid **and** they are peculiar.

         b. Relate strange mental experiences, reason in odd
             ways, and are difficult to get to know. None is of
             psychotic proportion.

         c. Manifest anxiety in social situations, have eccentric
             behavior, may be suspicious.

         d. Increased frequency of schizophrenia in first degree
             family members of persons who are schizotypal.

         e. E.g., the person who reports a "sixth sense",
             telekinetic and astral projection type experiences.

B. <u>Cluster B</u>: <u>Individuals are dramatic, erratic, and labile.</u>

   1. **Histrionic Personality Disorder:**

      a. Emotional instability (flighty); over-reactivity and dramatization; attention-seeking.

      b. Sexualize everything; except bed.

      c. Self-centered and vain; superficial; dependent.

      d. E.g., the 50 year old man who dresses like a 21 year old, goes to singles bars and tries to pick up 18 year olds with whom he is impotent.

   2. **Narcissistic Personality Disorder:**

      a. Usually symptom free and function well.

      b. Chronically unsatisfied due to constant needs for admiration.

      c. Believe selves to be "special persons" who are "<u>entitled</u>"; ideas of omnipotence; usually exploitative in interpersonal relationships.

      d. Grandiose, lacking in empathy and hypersensitive to evaluation by others.

      e. E.g., the supervisor who reacts to critical suggestion with vindictive retaliation. Uses anyone to own ends regardless of consequences to others.

   3. **Antisocial Personality Disorder:**

      a. Incapable of sufficient loyalty, so can't sustain a monogamous relationship for more than one year.

      b. No guilt; lies.

      c. Slow to learn from experience or punishment.

      d. Low frustration tolerance; can't delay gratification; reckless.

      e. Rationalization/blame others for difficulties.

      f. Grossly impaired parenting ability; can't hold a job.

      g. Frequent difficulty with the law.

h. <u>Very high familial distribution of this disorder and is more common in males.</u>

i. E.g., the unsuccessful criminal who ends up in trouble with the legal system.

4. **Borderline Personality Disorder:**

a. Show symptoms of schizophrenia but no history of a full psychotic episode in these individuals.

b. Have difficulties forming relationships, although frequently report the desire for such.

c. Display vagueness, pan-anxiety and pan-sexuality.

d. Lives are marked by instability in identity, mood and relationships.

e. Often self-mutilation.

f. Emotional lability and dyscontrol.

g. Have been known to have "micro-psychotic" episodes in which they deteriorate very rapidly into a blatantly psychotic condition with hallucinations, delusions, etc., for a period of one to two minutes. Reconstitute without assistance. Micro-psychotic episodes are precipitated by stress.

h. Splitting different people into categories of bad or good; or the same person is bad or good on different occasions. Sets people against each other.

i. E.g., the person who holds their hand in a flame in order to manipulate someone to do something the patient wants done.

C. <u>Cluster C:</u> <u>Individuals seem fearful, inhibited, and anxious.</u>

1. **Avoidant Personality Disorder:**

a. Very shy and hypersensitive with low self-esteem.

b. Have social discomfort, timid, and fear negative evaluation and embarrassment.

c. Would rather avoid personal contacts than face any potential social disapproval, even though they want personal involvement.

d. Often have anxiety and depression as accompaniments.

e. E.g., the person who walks down the street with their hand to their face so they don't see anyone else.

2. **Dependent Personality Disorder:**

a. Passive, unsure of self.

b. Tend to be loners who entirely depend on one or more people, and consequently can't be alone.

c. If relationship becomes threatened, deteriorate into anxiety and depression; so, go to great lengths to preserve relations in order to avoid feelings of abandonment.

d. Hurt by negative feedback.

e. E.g., the 35 year old person who lives at home with their parents and only socializes with the parents.

3. **Obsessive-Compulsive Personality Disorder:**

NOTE: This is different from the Obsessive Compulsive Disorder.

a. In this disorder, behaviors don't tend to bother the person but they **bother others**.

b. Excessive conformity and adherence to standards of conscience; overinhibited; overdutiful; unable to relax.

c. "Always right".

d. Have trouble making decisions and therefore being productive.

e. No generosity.

f. Pattern of perfectionism and inflexibility.

g. Poor (absent) interpersonal relations.

h. Always aware of their relative place on a dominance hierarchy.

i. More common in males.

j. E.g., the husband who insists the wife keep spices organized by the size and color of the container, not the content or alphabetic name of the spice.

4. **Passive-Aggressive Personality Disorder:**

   a. Inappropriate expression of one or more of the following: hostility, aggression, independence/ dependence, dominance/ submission.

   b. Procrastinators who rebel by doing nothing.

   c. Display passive resistance for adequate social and occupational performance.

   d. Won't do appropriate share of work.

   e. Scorns authority.

   f. E.g., the student who is always late for class and _never_ hands in assignments promptly.

III. **TREATMENT**

   A. Usually these patients come for therapy in one of two situations.

      1. Their behavior has produced some very negative consequences which they wish to avoid. E.g., the antisocial has been apprehended stealing something from someone and is attempting to avoid incarceration.

      2. The behavioral defense of the Personality Disorder is not working; and, the person is experiencing anxiety or depression. In this instance, they do not usually want to change the Personality Disorder, they want the therapist to help them return to thier previous pattern.

   B. Biologic/somatic interventions for the most part have proven to be relatively ineffective, except symptom relief and treatment for co-existing Axis I disorder.

   C. Long-term individual psychotherapy has proven somewhat successful, particularly when the therapist has very strong control of the patient's environment, e.g., the patient is directed by the court to be actively involved in psychotherapy. The most successful approaches seem to involve the following.

      1. The therapist should recognize these are very difficult patients who have had a lifetime of maladaptive behavior which is ego-syntonic. Therefore, they have little motivation for life-style change.

2. The therapist must set very clear and firm limits on the patients unacceptable behaviors.

3. Consequences of acting out (e.g., self destructive behavior, missing appointments, not paying the therapist's fees, etc.) should be clearly spelled out and followed the first and every time acting out occurs.

4. Give up messianic goals of "curing" the patient in a short period of time.

CHAPTER 10

ADJUSTMENT DISORDERS

I. DEFINITION

A. Acute maladaptive reactions to an identifiable psychosocial stress (or multiple stressors).

B. Occurs within three months of the stressor.

C. Extant for no more than six months after the stressor is relieved. If stressor continues, reaction can continue.

D. Symptoms may vary dramatically between individuals and within an individual from time to time.

    1. Impair social and occupational function

    2. Are "too much" reaction to the stressor.

E. Many think that any person can be brought to the point of an Adjustment Disorder if a stressor(s) is kept in place on a given individual long enough and with enough intensity.

II. TYPES (DSM-III-R)

A. Adjustment Disorder with Depressed Mood.

    1. The major symptoms that are seen are the depressive syndrome; crying and feelings of hopelessness, helplessness and worthlessness.

    2. E.g., a person who reacts to a job loss with a Protracted Depression Syndrome.

B. Adjustment Disorder with Anxious Mood.

    1. Patient presents with symptoms of "nervousness, worry, and jitteriness." Signs of anxiety are also present: e.g., tremor, excessive perspiration, etc..

    2. E.g., a person who reacts to a run-away child's behavior with marked anxiety.

C. Adjustment Disorder with Mixed Emotional Features.

    1. The individual may have signs of multiple emotional states such as depression, anxiety, anger, disgust, etc..

    2. E.g., a person who reacts to school failure with suicidal behavior and anxiety.

D. Adjustment Disorder with Disturbance of Conduct.

1. Instead of emotional expression, the person presents with behaviors in which there is a violation of the rights of others or of major age-appropriate societal norms and rules. E.g., delinquent behavior, violence, theft, irresponsibility, substance abuse, etc..

2. E.g., a person who reacts to the loss of a fiance' with substance abuse.

E. Adjustment Disorder with Mixed Disturbance of Emotions and Conduct.

1. Presents with both emotional symptoms and disturbance of conduct.

2. E.g., a person who reacts to a robbery with traffic violations and outbursts of crying.

F. Adjustment Disorder with Physical Complaints.

1. Instead of emotional or behavioral problems, the expression of the stressor is in physical symptoms, e.g., fatigue, headache, backache, or other aches and pains, that are not diagnosable as a physical disorder or condition.

2. E.g., the person who reacts to retirement with low back pain and muscle spasms.

G. Adjustment Disorder with Withdrawal

1. In this condition the person simply withdraws from social interaction with others. They do not manifest emotional or behavioral features other than the withdrawal. It appears to be withdrawal in order to "heal".

2. E.g., the person who reacts to a pets death by staying home with the blinds drawn.

H. Adjustment Disorder with Work (or Academic) Inhibition.

1. The person reacts to the stressor with an inhibition in work or academic functioning from a previous level of adequate functioning. In this situation there is frequently a mixture of anxiety and depression.

2. E.g., the person who reacts to discord with classmates by not going to school.

I. <u>Adjustment Disorder Not Otherwise Specified</u>

    1. If the person is clearly having an adjustment reaction to a specific stressor and they do not fit into one of the above categories, they are diagnosed here.

III. **TREATMENT**

    A. Psychotherapy and psycho-education is the treatment of choice. Therapy is focused on reducing the psychological impact of the stressor on the patient.

    B. Family/marital therapy is particularly indicated when the stressor is being brought by an identifiable person(s) who doesn't seem aware of the reaction their behavior is causing.

CHAPTER 11

PSYCHOLOGICAL FACTORS AFFECTING PHYSICAL CONDITIONS

I. **DEFINITION:**

   A. These are physical symptoms and changes in the physical structure of the body (signs) associated with mental factors. They can be an exacerbation of a physical condition, e.g. angina pain. Old term was Psychosomatic Disorders.

   B. Differentiate from Conversion Disorders on the following:

      1. These are controlled by the autonomic nervous system, while the Conversion Disorders predominantly involve portions of the body innervated by the voluntary nervous system or the special sense organs.

      2. The symptoms don't symbolize the psychological conflict like Conversion Disorders do. The person reacts in a given autonomic physiologic system with a symptom or symptoms that is (are) characteristic of that person, e.g., pre-ventricular contractions (PVC's) and gastric reflux.

      3. These reactions can produce tissue damage; Conversion Disorders characteristically do not. Might be GI tract ulcers, migraine headaches, hypertension, nausea and vomiting, etc..

II. **ETIOLOGY:** This is the epitome of the **Bio-Psycho-Social** Model of disease. That is:

   A. Biologic factors: e.g., hereditary predispositions or vulnerabilities, interact with--

   B. Psychological factors: e.g., optimistic versus pessimistic outlook, interact with--

   C. Social/environmental factors: e.g., being caught in a hopeless environmental setting like having to live in a socio-economically-deprived ghetto.

   D. The result then is dysfunction in one or more organ system of the body: e.g., dermatologic problems, respiratory problems, cardio-vascular difficulties, etc..

   It is significant that virtually all systems of the body can be negatively affected by psychological factors; and, many extant diseases (e.g., cancer) can be significantly impacted by psychological factors.

III. **TREATMENT**: the most effective treatments incorporate multi-modality intervention. The most effective treatments simultaneously address the:

  A. <u>Symptom</u>: e.g., peptic ulcer disease can be ameliorated with medications.

  B. <u>Stress or psychological factors</u>: e.g., allow the person to express the conflict/stress in the context of a safe setting (like the confidential confines of the professional's office); train the person to more realistically address stressful situations.

  Supportive psychotherapy is a major ingredient of coping with symptom complex involved.

  C. <u>Dysfunctional environment</u>: e.g., assist the person in effecting a realistic change in their life setting (obtain vocational rehabilitation assistance to improve the living situation); help the wife and the children of an abusive husband/father find other living arrangements or get them to a safe shelter where they are protected from further abuse.

CHAPTER 12

SEXUAL ISSUES AND DYSFUNCTIONS

I. SEXUAL DEVELOPMENT

A. Course of Development

1. **Sex or gender** refers to anatomy, physiology, and chromosomes. Sex chromosomes program differentiation of gonads into testes or ovaries.

   a. Embryonal gonad is influenced by material contained in sex chromosomes which leads to testes or ovaries to develop.

      - if testes develop they secrete testosterone (androgen).

      - without this testosterone, the reproductive system develops as female.

      - that is, the basic anatomical state of all fetuses is female. The addition of androgens (testosterone) during a "critical period" is necessary for a differentiation of male genitalia.

   b. In lower animals a sexually dimorphic nucleus is located in the hypothalamus.

      - If androgens are available prenatally, the hypothalamic cells become organized into a "male" pattern and at puberty "masculine" sexual behavior.

      - If androgens are absent prenatally the hypothalamic cells become organized into "female" patterns.

   c. Summary

      (1) Males: Apparently the presence of androgen programs differentiation of external genitalia, the hypothalamus and other CNS structures into masculine activities, structure, and function.

      (2) Females: PROBABLY the absence of androgen results in external genitalia, programming the hypothalamus and other CNS structures into female activities, structure, and function.

2. **Birth:** The person is born (hopefully) with external genitalia and CNS structures that are fairly well defined.

3. **Gender Identity:** Refers to sexual roles such as masculinity or femininity. The **feeling** of "Am I a male or a female?" Established by age 2 or 3. The **private experience** of sex role. After birth: the response of significant others continues to assign the gender identity.

   Depends on:

   a. Gender development.

   b. Well developed secondary sex characteristics.

   c. Normal endocrine function.

   d. Significant others' expectations of sex role.

   e. Language

4. **Gender identification:** the masculine or feminine behavior of the person. Learned from role models while growing up, at home, preschool, kindergarten, and grade school. Usually in place by puberty. This is the **public expression** of sex role.

   Sexual feelings and behavior are shaped by:

   a. Gender identity

   b. Socially imposed rules, values and standards.

   c. Early life experiences.

   d. Presence of a clear role model.

   e. Here and now cues and opportunities.

NOTE: Gender, Gender Identity and Gender Identification may match or not. E.g., individual can have male genitalia, a feminine identity, and male identification. Would look male anatomically and behaviorally, but feel like a female.

II.   **SEXUAL DYSFUNCTIONS**

    A. Sexual Aversion Disorder

       1. Person has no interest in any genital sexual contact with a partner.

       2. Etiology is from a wide variety of sources that are environmental, psychological, interpersonal, physical, medical, etc. in nature.

       3. **Treatment:** if the person complains of the situation, resolution of the etiologic factors is the goal.

    B. Male Erectile Disorder

       1. Inability to erect the penis, and little if any pleasure in sexual activity.

       2. Most often due to performance anxiety, fatigue, or stress. Other biologic causes: early undiagnosed diabetes; low androgen level; estrogenic medication; hepatic problems; toxicity on alcohol, narcotics, or sedative-hypnotics; neurological diseases; MS; tumors (structural or hormone secreting); operations (e.g. prostatectomy), alpha adrenergic blockade.

       3. Must differentiate primary versus secondary.

          a. Primary: has never had the ability, or has been able to erect on rare occasions.

          b. Secondary: was able and has now lost the ability.

       4. Rarely is this dysfunction 100% in a given man. Usually can perform under certain circumstance.

       5. **Treatment:** Resolution of the underlying condition.

          a. In primary issues, probably psychotherapy is indicated.

          b. In secondary, is oriented to isolating the etiologic condition and reversing it if possible.

          c. If desire is present and through physiologic studies it is determined that there is no physical ability to perform, penile implants can be done to give erectile function.

C. Female Arousal Disorder

   1. No vaginal lubrication or labial injection, coupled with minimal pleasure.

   2. Etiologies similar to that of males. Some find sexuality repugnant or a "duty" (early training?).

   3. **Treatment:** resolution of underlying factors. If psychogenic in nature, then psychotherapy is major intervention.

D. Inhibited Male Orgasm

   1. Difficulty having intravaginal orgasm. Can have orgasm to other activity such as masturbation, fellatio, etc.

   2. Etiologies may be psychological, interpersonal, medical, toxic in nature.

   3. **Treatment:** Resolution of underlying etiology.

      a. If psychogenic, psychotherapy is indicated.

      b. If interpersonal, couples therapy is the treatment of choice.

      c. If physiologic, medical or toxic, medical attention is warranted.

E. Inhibited Female Orgasm (Anorgasmia)

   1. Female cannot have orgasm from any source.

   2. Etiologies similar to males.

      a. Psychologically, the ability to have orgasm in females is very highly correlated with the extent to which she feels she can trust her partner.

   3. **Treatment:** Similar to males. But it should be noted that there are severe and extreme restrictions on females that are not placed on males. Therefore, the probability that a more intrapsychic etiology is present should be considered.

F. Premature Ejaculation

   1. Regular extravaginal ejaculation occurs when intercourse is being attempted; or, lack of voluntary control.

2. **Etiology:** never learned control techniques, or may be the expression of an interpersonal conflict.

3. **Treatment:** Easily treated with the "Squeeze Technique." At times of unwanted ejaculation, the head of the penis is squeezed tightly to abort the ejaculation. Voluntary control is gained through this procedure.

G. Dyspareunia:

1. Painful intercourse for the female.

2. **Etiology:**

    a. Usually physiologic in nature (e.g. tipped uterus, infection, inflammation, depth penetration). Occurs in males as function of infection, irritation, etc..

    b. If the female is inhibited about responding, she may suppress the human sexual response cycle, inhibit the excitement phase and create a vaginal environment in which friction is painful.

3. **Treatment:**

    a. Resolve the underlying physical problem.

    b. If psychogenic, psychotherapy and education is indicated.

H. Vaginismus:

1. Strong contractions of the walls of the vagina. Impossible to insert a finger or penis.

2. **Etiology**

    a. Possibly classically conditioned response to underlying dyspareunia.

    b. May reflect unconscious inhibited responding.

3. **Treatment**

    a. If dyspareunia is resolved, in vivo desensitization with graduated vaginal dilators is helpful.

    b. If is psychogenic, psychotherapy is the treatment of choice.

III. ADULT SEXUAL DISORDERS

A. <u>Gender Dysphoria</u> (Transsexuality):

1. **Definition:** The feeling in a biologically normal person of being a member of the opposite sex (Gender Identity reversal).

2. **Etiology:** Unknown. Many think it is a biologic variation secondary to altered physiologic processes at conception and\or during intrauterine development.

3. **Treatment:** Seek surgical correction of external appearance to be consistent with internal feelings.

   a. <u>Surgery is not organ transplant.</u> Is restructuring genitals. E.g. creating vaginal labia and vagina in biologic males; creating a penis, scrotum, testes in biologic females.

   b. Long involved process of screening and conversion.

      (1) Requirements/precautions before operation:

         (a) Psychiatric evaluation to establish diagnosis. Requires 1-2 years. To eliminate person with other mental disorders being inappropriately managed.

         (b) Live/work in other sex role one year before operation.

         (c) Hormone treatments during that or following year.

   c. Approximately 10% of those presenting receive final surgery.

   d. There has been no long term psychotherapeutic success in reversing the gender dysphoria of a person who is a true transsexual.

B. <u>Paraphilias</u>

1. **Definition:** recurrent intense sexual urges and sexually arousing fantasies generally involving either (1) nonhuman subjects, (2) the suffering or humiliation of oneself or one's partner (not merely simulated), or (3) children or other nonconsenting persons.

These also generally include a criterion that the behavior more or less interferes with the capacity for reciprocal, affectionate sexual activity. There are nine subtypes.

a. Pedophilia:

    (1)   Sexual preference by an adult person for a minor child.

    (2)   More reported in males, but recent data suggest females also have high rates of sexual abuse of children.

    (3)   Usually fondling: vaginal or anal penetration, while not common is not rare.

    (4)   **Incest** as a special form of Pedophilia

        (a)   Sexual relations between two persons who are too closely related by blood to marry. The definition is often extended to step-parent step-children dyads. Laws concerning incest vary among States.

        (b)   Most common form of incest is probably siblings. This is most common in families in which children share the same bedroom and poor parental supervision. Usually ignored as "exploration."

                The most common **reported** form is father-daughter (stepfather-daughter, boyfriend-daughter) incest. Mother-son incest occurs. Was believed the mother had awareness of father-daughter incest; and, through silence or discounting daughter's report, condoned it. New data suggest mothers are frequently unaware.

        (c)   Reported to be almost **universally taboo.**

        (d)   Kinsey researchers reported the male incest offender is ineffectual, often drunk, often unemployed man who is deprived of sex. Once the incest taboo is broken, they continue. **Availability and ease of access are the motivating forces. 45% are under the influence of alcohol at the time of offense.**

Now known to occur in all Socio-Economic-Strata with a wide diversity of persons and motivations.

    (5)   **Etiology:** shrinking away from mature adult reciprocal relations where risk of performance evaluation is present. Some report the desire for a "pure (virginal)" sex partner.

b. <u>Exhibitionism</u>:

    (1)   Is a male prosecuted condition. I.e., females who display their genitals to males are not arrested.

    (2)   The individual has the compulsion to exhibit penis to a child or an adult (or both) for purpose of sexual gratification.

            No desire for further sexual contact; but intent is to elicit a response (e.g., startle) from the other person.

    (3)   Psychologically it is assumed that the act is an attempt to reassure the self that the penis is still present after the person has encountered a "castrating" event, e.g., being "put down" at work.

    (4)   Exhibitionists report sexual arousal while they are anticipating the event; and they usually derive sexual release by masturbation during or after they have exposed themselves.

    (5)   Often married and live stable lives.

c. <u>Voyeurism</u>:

    (1)   Only prosecuted in males.

    (2)   A sexual situation in which witnessing certain events has become a sexual need and slowly becomes the major outlet for sexual gratification.

d. <u>Fetishism</u>:

    (1)   Person is sexually aroused by an object, not a person: e.g., shoes, pantyhose, women's handkerchiefs, etc..

(2) Uses the object in sexual activity--usually masturbation. May want sexual partner to wear or use the object during a sexual episode.

(3) Etiology: probably object was associated with a loved person or a sexually stimulating event early in childhood.

(4) Mainly a male prosecuted disorder.

e. <u>Frotteurism</u>:

(1) Sexual stimulation and/or gratification by rubbing the body against an unsuspecting person. E.g., standing in a crowded area and rubbing the genital against the buttocks of another person.

(2) Mainly a male prosecuted disorder.

f. <u>Sexual Masochism</u>:

(1) The person wishes pain, suffering, and/or humiliation to be inflicted on themself for sexual excitement.

(2) Etiology may be early experiences where person was exposed to sensuality and pain simultaneously. E.g., parent placing child face down on the parent's knees and spanking the child. Child's genitals stimulated by parent's knees.

Others report they desire the pain "in order to feel", i.e., they are so inhibited regarding sexual feelings that it takes inordinate amounts of stimulation to overcome the inhibition.

g. <u>Sexual Sadism</u>:

(1) Pain, suffering, humiliation inflicted on another for sexual excitement.

(2) Sometimes kills victim after the torture has been inflicted.

(3) Many have co-existent other serious psychiatric disorders often of psychotic proportions.

h. <u>Transvestic Fetishism</u>:

    (1)   A fetishistic, pleasurable, sporadic cross-dressing in a biologically normal man who doesn't question he is a male.

    (2)   Usually married, heterosexual, and has children.

    (3)   As opposed to fetishism, entire wardrobes may be involved.

    (4)   Cross-dressing enhances the sexual excitement.

i. <u>Other conditions</u>:

    (1)   **Telephone scatologia** (lewdness): "Obscene telephone calls" where the caller is attempting to get a reaction from the person called. May be related to Exhibitionism.

    (2)   **Necrophilia:** The individual has sexual contact and gratification with dead bodies. Many have a co-existent psychotic level psychiatric disorder.

    (3)   **Partialism** (exclusive focus on one part of the body, e.g. toes.)

    (4)   **Zoophilia:** The preference for animal sexual contact.

    (5)   **Coprophilia:** The person wishes to defecate on a partner; or to be defecated on by the partner for sexual stimulation and/or gratification.

    (6)   **Urophilia:** The person wishes to urinate on or be urinated on for sexual stimulation and/or gratification. Also called a "golden shower".

    (7)   **Klismaphilia:** The person either gives or gets enemas as a part of sexual stimulation and/or gratification.

C. <u>Treatment of the Paraphilias</u>

1. Generally the paraphilias require long-term, insight-oriented psychotherapy.

2. Sometimes this is coupled with more behaviorally oriented sex therapy to allow the person to be functional in situations outside the paraphilic condition.

3. If there is co-morbidity, addressing control of the other psychiatric condition is necessary.

CHAPTER 13

SPECIAL PROBLEMS OF CHILDREN

I. GENERAL ISSUES

A. Children show problems of adjustment as they mature, but typically they develop out of these. Some become disorders.

B. Most of the disorders of adults can occur in children (e.g., schizophrenia, affective disorders, etc.).

C. The notable exceptions are the Axis II diagnoses which are not diagnosed in persons under 18 years of age.

D. However there are disorders of childhood that are differentiated from those of adults.

II. SPECIAL DISORDERS OF CHILDHOOD: GROUPED INTO 5 CATEGORIES.

A. Category 1: Developmental Disorders

1. Mental Retardation

    a. Definition: Composed of at least 3 variables

    (1) **Organic**: structural/physiologic problems. E.g., microencephaly; phenylketonuria; Down's Syndrome (Trisomy 21); mercury, lead encephalopathy; metabolic issues (e.g., cretinism; Leach-Nyhan Syndrome, with self mutilation like chewing lips and fingers); thalidomide; irradiation; and possible psychoactive drug exposure or ingestion during pregnancy.

    Infections during the first trimester of pregnancy: bacterial meningitis, congenital syphilis, viral encephalitis, tuberculosis meningitis, cytomegalovirus, rubella mycoplasma, toxoplasmosis etc..

    (2) **Functional**: "disability" arises from individual's psychological reaction to limitation imposed on function by organic impairment or by psychological and/or social forces.

    (3) **Social**: special roles assigned to the retarded individual within the family, peer groups, schools, society, etc.. The manner in which primary impairment and functional disability

alter socially expected performance determines the degree of "mental handicap." **Families tend to socialize less if there is a retarded child in the home.**

b. Poverty and lower socio-economic class decrease access to medical care during and after pregnancy, resulting in increased prematurity, poor nutrition, more infections, and deprivation. All contribute to an increase in incidence of mental retardation (particularly mild retardation).

c. More diagnosed in males. May reflect the observation that male offspring have more difficulty with the birth process.

d. Diagnosis for both males and females is usually at school entry.

e. IQ Scores and Classification (DSM-III-R):

    (1)   Mild: 50-55 to about 70. Educable
    (2)   Moderate: 35-40 to 50-55. Trainable.
    (3)   Severe: 20-25 to 35-40. Custodial.
    (4)   Profound: below 20-25. Custodial.

f. Onset before age 18. If occurs after 18, considered to be dementia.

2. **Autistic Disorder** (Pervasive Developmental Disorder)

a. <u>First major characteristic</u>. Kanner (1943): inability to relate self in the ordinary manner to people and situations from the beginning of life. Don't withdraw from previous existing participation with others (as in the schizophrenias).

    (1)   Fascination for objects while having poor or absent relationships to people.

    (2)   Do not respond to mother's affection or tenderness.

b. <u>Second major characteristic</u>: failure to use language for communication. Often thought to be deaf since do not respond to communications. Can be differentiated from deafness by auditory evoked potential.

c. <u>Third major characteristic</u>: an anxiously obsessive desire for sameness. They display fear of new patterns.

d. Very marked restriction in repertoire of activities and interests. Sometimes display bizarre behaviors e.g., head banging and rocking. Don't play normally with other kids.

e. Most have a co-existing diagnosis of mental retardation.

f. Treatment modalities for these children include behavior modification techniques (food and smiling rewards for behaviors desired to appear). More traditional psychodynamic therapy also used. Important prognostic milestone is if the child has useful language by the age of 5.

g. Long-term follow-up: even if have become somewhat socialized in a "normal" way, as adult tend to be loners and seek solitary occupations.

h. The etiology of this disorder is not known. The incidence is approximately 1 per 2,500 children. Have found correlates of neurologic dysfunction.

3. **Specific Developmental Disorders**

a. <u>Academic Skills Disorders</u>

(1) **Reading.** <u>Dyslexia</u>: defined as a perceptual problem which can occur in any sensory modality (usually in the visual and auditory senses) and which interferes with learning.   Characterization:

(a) Above average intelligence, vocabulary and social development. Male to female is 10:1. Usually left handed. Again may reflect birth process difficulties for males.

(b) Visual perceptual defect

i) Position in space difficulties; inability to differentiate mirror letters, e.g. "b" and "d"; "m" and "w", "p" and "q", etc..

ii) Foreground/background reversals: If looking at chalkboard with writing on it, alternately keys visual perception on the white lines and then the spaces formed by the letters.

iii) Form constancy: Inability to equate two items that differ in minor characteristics but are basically the same. E.g., "dog" is not recognized as the same as "DOG"

iv) Visual motor coordination: problems for males in athletics since cannot catch a ball when thrown to him.

(c) Auditory perceptual defect: similar phenomenon here to the visual counterpart.

(d) Etiology: believed to be brain dysfunction, maturational lag in brain development, and/or heredity.

(2) **Arithmetic**

(3) **Expressive/receptive language**

(4) **Articulation**

(5) **Writing**

(6) **Coordination**

D. Category 2: Disruptive Behavior Disorders

1. **Attention-Deficit Hyperactivity Disorder**

a. Definition: characterized by overactivity, restlessness, short attention span, & distractibility. It is almost unceasing and is not outgrown (if at all) until late in development. Data suggest 5-10% of the school population suffers from the disorder.

b. Course of the disturbance:

(1) Infant often unusually active, develops rapidly, sleeps little, and cries frequently.

(2) Problem heightened when reaches the age for socialization and formal education. Literally cannot sit still long enough to learn.

         (3)   Oversensitivity to stimulation makes it impossible to attend to one stimulus at a time, but is also unable to reject other sensory stimuli coming into CNS.

         (4)   Usually quite bright; rarely retarded. This in turn leads to disapproval from adults who do not understand the behavior. "You could do better than that if you'd just try. You're very bright."

c. Diagnosis is made primarily from the patient's history, but transient neurological signs, EEG changes, and lowered seizure thresholds have occasionally been found. **Differentiate these children from those who are mentally retarded, hearing impaired, or emotionally disturbed.**

d. Treatment usually consists of daily doses of CNS stimulants which have a "paradoxical" effect on hyperkinetic children.

e. It has been said that the disorder is outgrown between 12 and 18 and the medication is discontinued. This finding is questioned today. Emotional problems which may have developed secondary to hyperkinesis must be dealt with therapeutically from a psychological standpoint.

2. **Conduct Disorder**

a. Repetitive and persistent pattern of conduct (lasting at least 6 months) whose core symptom is that the basic rights of others and social norms are violated. Physical aggression (e.g. rape), breaking and entering crimes, cruelty to animals and stealing are common.

         (1)   Solitary aggressive type where the child acts alone with aggressive violation.

         (2)   Group type where the violations occur in the context of a group/gang.

         (3)   Undifferentiated type is where the child has both solitary and group involvement.

         (4)   Often from homes where adults are diagnosed as Antisocial Personality Disorder.

b. Juvenile Delinquency: May be a conduct disorder, but is a legal label not a psychiatric diagnosis. Usually includes a background of:

   (1) Parent separation or severe neglect/abuse/incest.

   (2) Psychological disabilities, e.g. dyslexia.

   (3) Feelings of (physical) inferiority.

   (4) Some reports of EEG abnormality (positive spiking).

   (5) Includes a complex of aggressive/destructive behaviors that are externally directed. May be a "rejection of rejecters."

   (6) **"Runaways"** are frequently classified as Juvenile Delinquents and sometimes as Conduct Disorders. They often have a history of victimization by incest, family violence, and/or restrictive parents.

   Over time, runaways tend to become involved in violence, drugs, promiscuity, and venereal disease, particularly if not returned to their home and/or the home conditions have not changed.

3. **Oppositional Defiant Disorder**

   a. Characterized by negativistic, hostile and defiant behaviors (blames others, swears, vindictive, deliberately annoys others, etc.).

   b. Generally do not violate the rights of others.

C. Category 3: Anxiety Disorders of Childhood or Adolescence

1. **Separation Anxiety Disorder**

   a. Excessive anxiety concerning separation from attachment figure. Includes unrealistic worry, school refusal, repeated nightmares about separation, and excessive signs of distress on separation. May get to the point of panic.

    b. School Phobia is a special type of Separation Anxiety Disorder.

       (1)   Considered an emergency equivalent to childhood suicide.

       (2)   Etiology usually lies in the mother/child relationship where the child fears that the mother will not be home or will be ill/dead when the child returns. Sometimes onset after mother has been ill.

       (3)   Other causes are peer abuse, fear of teachers and authority, fear of failure.

       (4)   Distinguish from truancy where the parents don't know child is missing school.

       (5)   Usually treated by insisting the child go to school, but allowing the child to call home between classes for reassurance the parent is still there.

2. Avoidant Disorder

    a. Painful shyness and withdrawal from unfamiliar people, leading to interference in social functioning with peers.

    b. Must last for at least 6 months, and the child must be at least 2 1/2 years old.

3. Overanxious Disorder

    a. Generalized and persistent anxiety or worry, not related to separation from significant others (e.g. unrealistic worry about future or past events, etc.).

    b. Because this symptom complex can occur in normal children, the finding must last at least 6 months in order to establish the diagnosis.

D. Category 4: Physical Disorders

1. Eating Disorders

    a. <u>Anorexia nervosa</u>: do not maintain an appropriate body weight, fear of gaining weight.

       (1)   No organic cause for the weight loss

      (2)   Weight loss of at least 25% of body weight

      (3)   Usually adolescent female, accompanied by amenorrhea. Can be male.

      (4)   Disturbed body image where **believes** is overweight. Frequently the central psychodynamic core is a sexual identity issue where the young person doesn't "want to grow up". Maintenance of thinness gives prepubertal image.

      (5)   About 1/3 had a minor weight problem and significant others reinforced weight loss.

      (6)   Tends to run in families.

      (7)   Recent data suggest a dopamine, serotonin and norepinephrine component.

b. <u>Bulimia Nervosa</u>

      (1)   A "gorge and purge" syndrome

      (2)   Gorging done in a discrete time period, and person feels has no control. May be planned and usually high calorie foods are eaten.

      (3)   A number of person with Bulimia will steal food.

      (4)   Purging usually done through induced vomiting and sometimes with laxatives. May take on aspects of relieving guilt for gorging.

                NOTE: The constant vomiting results in erosion of teeth due to hyperacidity in the mouth.

      (5)   Underlying characteristics are similar to anorexia nervosa.

c. <u>Pica</u>: eating non-nutritive substances (e.g. paint, plaster, hair, dirt, sand, pebbles, etc.) for at least one month; **not during pregnancy.**

d. <u>Rumination disorder of infancy</u>

      (1)   Partially digested food is brought into the mouth, rechewed, and reswallowed.

      (2)   Usually appears between 3 and 12 months of age.

2. **Tic Disorders**

   a. <u>Tourette's Disorder</u>:

     (1)   Multiple motor and one or more vocal tics (e.g. coprolalia, nonverbal sounds like barking, grunts, etc.).

     (2)   Occur multiple times during the day.

     (3)   Lifelong.

     (4)   Possibly genetic.

     (5)   Treatment is with antipsychotics in low dosages.

   b. <u>Chronic Motor or Vocal Tic Disorder</u>: Motor or vocal tics; present > one year.

   c. <u>Transient Tic Disorder</u>: Tics present < 12 months.

3. **Elimination Disorders**

   a. <u>Enuresis</u>: In non-retarded, non-brain dysfunctional children, after age 3, especially if diurnal as well as nocturnal wetting. Males> females. Can be intentional.

     (1)   Forms

       (a)   <u>Primary</u>: child has never achieved bladder control. **Usually same sex parent was bed wetter.** Probably due to deep Stage 4 sleep where full bladder cues can't awaken the child. Occurs most often in the first 1/3 of the night.

       (b)   <u>Secondary</u>: child achieved bladder control, begins wetting again usually after identifiable psychic trauma: e.g., birth of sibling, a move, etc..

     (2)   Rarely occurs as only symptom; often associated with fire setting, impulsiveness, delinquency, etc..

     (3)   Rule out physical cause first; found in < 5-10%.

     (4)   Treatment: Behavior Modification with bell and pad; awaken child in the first 1/3 of the night

to void; medications to lighten Stage 4 sleep; restrict fluids after 6:00 p.m.; etc..

    b. Encopresis

        (1) Child repeatedly has bowel movements in places that are age inappropriate.

        (2) May be purposeful.

        (3) Once per month for at least 6 months, and child's mental and chronological age is at least 4 years.

E. Category 5: Gender Identity Disorders

  1. **Gender Identity Disorder of Childhood**

    a. Persistent and intense distress in a child about their biologic sex; and a desire to be or insistence that they are of the other sex. Won't accept anatomic body or function of their biologic sex.

    b. Females do not like female clothing.

    c. Males want to dress like a female and involve self in activities that are clearly feminine.

  2. **Transsexualism**

    a. After puberty, the child has wanted for at least two years to be rid of own sex characteristics and get those of opposite gender. Uncomfortable with assigned sex.

    b. Variant: person is uncomfortable with assigned sex; cross-dresses not for sexual excitement; and has no wish to be rid of primary or secondary sex characteristics.

F. General Notes on Childhood Disorders

  1. Neurologic dysfunction assessed through developmental delay.

  2. Usually measured through perceptual deficits and behavioral deviance.

  3. "Emotional disturbance" can be the cause or the effect of behavioral concomitants, e.g. short attention span.

III. **TREATMENT**

A. Behavior modification has been invaluable in addressing many basic childhood disorders, e.g. bed wetting, encopresis, etc..

B. Learning disabilities: special <u>educational</u> techniques have been developed to address the specific dysfunctions.

C. The field of psychopharmacology in children is just beginning to reach maturity. The area of childhood depression is where medications are under intensive study.

CHAPTER 14

SPECIAL ISSUES IN PSYCHIATRY

I. SLEEP DISORDERS

   A. Sleep:

      1. Stages and EEG equivalents: one complete cycle (Stages 1, 2, 3, and 4 and REM) lasts an average of 90 minutes.

      2. Structures in the lower pons and medulla are responsible for initiating or maintaining sleep through synchronization of cortical rhythms. Presumably act through inhibition of the midbrain reticular system. Cortex isn't necessary for sleep.

         a. Stage 1: Low voltage-mixed frequency but most predominant is Theta (4-8 cps). (Similar to experienced meditators.)

         b. Stage 2: Between 1 and 3 and 4 (Spindles 12-14/second here, and random spikes.)

         c. Stages 3 and 4: Slow wave -- mainly Delta (less than 4 cps). High amplitude. Very deep sleep.

            Stages 1, 2, 3, and 4 are sometimes referred to as non-REM sleep.

         d. REM (rapid eye movement):

            (1)   Background EEG same as Stage 1 except bursts of lateral REM.

            (2)   Behavioral concomitants: a) vivid **visual dreams** like hallucinations. Non-visual dreams occur in other stages and resemble thoughts running through mind; b) **erections** in men and vasocongestion in women; c) **torso muscles** in state of total relaxation except for some finger,toe, limb twitches. Maybe facial grimace.

            (3)   In the autonomic nervous system, all measures except electrodermal activity are at their highest and lowest producing the greatest variability.

            (4)   In REM the lateral geniculate of the thalamus receives volleys of information from the pons. From the thalamus the information travels to the cortex. Another path goes from the pons to

the medulla and spinal cord. Nerve tissue
shows peak growth patterns with such
stimulation.

e. At all age groups after two years of age, <u>REM
constitutes about 20-25% of sleep</u>. Early in
infancy REM constitutes between 50% (age 1-3
months) and 40% (3-5 months) of sleep.

3. **Sleep correlates:**

a. Daytime wakefulness is more dependent upon
uninterrupted periods of sleep than total amount.

b. Sleep deprivation has a cumulative effect.

c. Age issues

(1) Sleep becomes progressively fragmented over the
course of a lifetime in that there is an
increase in the amount of waking time and the
number of awakenings after sleep onset.

(2) The percent of REM is highest in infants.

(3) Children: rarely awaken in the night and get
more REM in the last 2\3 of the night.

(4) Young adults get deep sleep early on with less
later in the night. REM increases as the night
goes on.

(5) In the elderly there is an equal distribution
of REM throughout the night; however, the major
problem is an increased number of awakenings
and a decrease in slow wave sleep. This
results in lighter sleep with more awakenings.

d. Deep sleep is associated with serotonin levels; and
wakefulness is associated with norepinephrine levels.

e. With sedative-hypnotic medication and alcohol, REM is
reduced; but in the chronic users on withdrawal, one
sees a rebound phenomenon with more than average REM.

4. **Unusual behavioral sleep states and the sleep cycle.**

a. <u>Sleep walking (somnambulism)</u>:

(1) 1-6% of population

(2) Males more than females

      (3)   Occurs in NON REM period

b. <u>Night terrors</u>:

      (1)   More frequent in children

      (2)   Characterized by anxiety, high ANS discharge, motility, verbalizations

      (3)   Stage 4 concomitant

      (4)   Not remembered the next day

      (5)   Upsets others because of the terror

c. <u>Narcolepsy</u>:

      (1)   Sudden irresistible sleep.

      (2)   Is rapid and instantaneous onset of REM sleep.

      (3)   Cataplexy: sudden loss of muscle tone with emotion. Occurs in 66-95% of narcoleptics.

      (4)   Recent data suggest may be an auto-immune disorder.

      (5)   May affect as many as 250,000 Americans.

      (6)   Treatment: take naps during the day; budget time; stimulant medication for the narcolepsy and tricyclic antidepressants for the cataplexy (suppresses REM).

d. <u>Nightmares</u>: During REM.

e. <u>Insomnia</u>: Correlated with depression; and have less REM.

f. <u>Enuresis</u>: (See Chapter 13)

      (1)   Non-REM

      (2)   Stage 4, 2, or 1

      (3)   Occurs in the first 1/3 of the night

II.   ACQUIRED IMMUNO-DEFICIENCY SYNDROME (AIDS)

A. The Changing Face of the AIDS Epidemic

1. Initially the majority of persons in the United States who had AIDS were homosexual males and the second largest group were IV drug users.

2. Presently this group represents only a bit over 50% of new cases; and women of child bearing years is becoming the leading demographic group. Many of these have been infected by their IV drug using male companions.

3. It is feared that due to sexual activity, drug use and poor education about alternatives and safer sex practices, the epidemic will spread to the teen-age group.

B. The Issues of Confidentiality

1. Potential Social Consequences

a. Loss of job and therefore health insurance.

b. Loss of living space: e.g., may be thrown out of apartment, etc..

c. Ostracism from social supports: e.g., school, church, etc.

2. Does society have a right to know the identity of persons with the virus?

a. Should HIV+ patients be known to their health care providers?

b. Should HIV+ health care workers be known to their patients?

C. Support System

1. Family and friends provide the vast majority of support for the infected and ill patient.

2. Access to medical care is limited by geographic concerns, financial availability and the relative ambulatory condition of the patient.

D. The Continuum of the Infection

1. The following "guestimates" are based on group data and represents the current scenario. This may change dramatically relatively quickly as new treatment methods are established.

2. **YEARS**

```
0---------0.5----------------------10-------13/15
EXPOSURE   SEROCONVERSION           AIDS        DEATH
```

3. Seroconversion is usually found after about 6 months post inoculation with the virus.

4. Note, people with AIDS do not represent the greatest risk for sexually transmitted AIDS. They are often too sick to be interested in sexual activity.

   People who are HIV+ and asymptomatic are the greatest risk for transmission because they often don't know, they feel healthy and they look healthy.

E. Psychological Issues

1. If the patient is HIV+, often enters the death and dying sequence of Denial, Anger, Bargaining, Sadness and Acceptance.

2. The quiet years after the person knows they are HIV positive often provokes feelings of being a walking time bomb and therefore much anxiety.

   Often persons in this stage show more distress than those with full blown AIDS.

3. The Onset of AIDS raises questions of:

   a. What's left?

   b. How soon is this going to kill me?

   c. What am I going to do until I die? "Living versus dying with AIDS.

F. "Safer Sex":   core and central issue is to not exchange body fluids. HIV is not spread by general social contact.

G. Death issues: Suicide as an option. Most have suicidal thoughts and don't act on them.

H. Psychiatric Issues.

   1. Primary Psychiatric Conditions

      a. Dementia: Occurs in about 2/3 of AIDS patients. Many times it is the early presenting symptom.

   2. Secondary Psychiatric Conditions

      a. Anxiety Reactions: Panic attacks, agitation, insomnia, anorexia, tachycardia.

      b. Depressive Syndrome

III. GERIATRIC PSYCHIATRY

A. Some statistical data:

   1. 4-5% of the persons >65 years of age live in institutions. Percent increases with each decade.

   2. 65%-80% of older persons live with someone else.

   3. 85% of elderly have one or more chronic health conditions.

B. Physiologic State

   1. In the aging process, humans lose about 50,000 neurons per day.

   2. Ventricles expand.

   3. Cerebral oxygen consumption falls.

   4. Formation of plaques increases.

   5. EEG abnormalities increase.

C. Major Psychiatric Disorders

   1. Alzheimer's Disease

      a. Correlated with pathology in the ACH system. Exact etiology unknown at this time.

      b. Brain imaging studies have repeatedly demonstrated deterioration in the posterior temporal-parietal areas.

c. The three phase manifestation:

  (1) <u>Tendency toward forgetfulness</u>: for names, places, and appointments. Show a joking anxiety about it.

  (2) <u>Confusional phase</u>: Memory for recent events severely impaired; memory for remote events often intact. Earlier Phase I anxiety is replaced by denial.

  (3) <u>Dementia phase</u>: severe disorientation; remote memory loss is added to the recent memory loss; concrete; no new learning; easily confused with environmental changes; eventually become apathetic; cannot care for self.

2. **Depression (Pseudodementia)**

  a. Major Depressive Disorder in the elderly person which is mistaken for a Dementia.

  b. Suicide is a very real risk in these persons.

3. **Anxiety**

  a. High rates as person begins to fear environmental invasion. Don't feel safe when alone.

  b. Anxiety connected with progressive loss of function and fear of the consequences (e.g., being placed in a nursing home).

  c. Fear of becoming a burden often results in suicide.

4. **Sleep Disorders in the Elderly**

  a. In the elderly there is an equal distribution of REM throughout the night.

  b. The major problem is an increased number of awakenings and a decrease in slow wave sleep. This results in lighter sleep with more awakenings.

  c. The elderly may try to self medicate with alcohol which further disrupts the sleep cycle.

  d. Very likely to request sleeping medications which are **ALL** addictive.

5. **Substance abuse**

   a. Alcoholism: as person becomes more isolated from social interchange with the world, alcohol consumption may increase.

   b. Iatrogenic: e.g., sedative-hypnotic addiction secondary to sleep problems; narcotic addiction secondary to pain from physical debilitation.

   c. "Accidental": e.g., when one tablet of sedative hypnotic no longer works (secondary to tolerance effects), the person doubles the previous dose.

6. **Delirium in the Elderly**

   a. Iatrogenic: most common cause is multiple medications from different health providers who are unaware of what others are prescribing.

IV. **LEGAL ASPECTS OF PSYCHIATRY**

A. <u>Expert Witness</u>

1. Can draw a conclusion from data which is presented to him. Therefore can have an "opinion" about certain issues involved in a given case.

2. Very frequently called upon to address the issue of an "Insanity" plea. <u>Note: Insanity is a legal term, it is not a psychiatric one.</u>

3. The Psychiatrist as an expert witness who can draw conclusions is associated with many of the following issues.

B. <u>Competency to Stand Trial</u>. Psychiatrist often asked to establish a persons competency to start trial. The psychiatrist's opinion is based on answering the following questions: Is the patient able to:

1. Understand nature of the charges?

2. Understand the possible penalties?

3. Understand the legal issues and procedures?

4. Work with the attorney?

5. Participate rationally in his own defense?

C. Informed Consent-**Adult**. Because of the apparent irreversibility of some effects of psychiatric intervention (e.g., tardive dyskinesia), the Psychiatrist must always determine if the patient understands:

   1. Reason for treatment.

   2. What is being prescribed.

   3. What probable outcomes are.

   4. What side effects are known to occur (e.g., Tardive Dyskinesia).

   5. Alternate treatments.

D. Informed Consent-**Parents**. If the patient is a child, then the parents or the appropriate guardian must give informed consent for the child. To do this:

   1. The parents must be told everything listed in C. above.

   2. The parents must give permission.

   3. If they won't give permission and the child's life is threatened, the courts can overrule the parents.

E. Informed consent when the patient cannot provide it. If the patient is too mentally disturbed to give their informed consent:

   1. A court appointed conservator or an attorney-in-fact can be designated with a "Durable Power of Attorney for Health Care."

   2. Immediate family members or close friends can be surrogate decision makers.

   3. If surrogate decision makers disagree; physician should continue to treat until a decision is reached or a conservator is appointed by the courts.

   4. If known, the patient's wishes take priority over other's.

   5. Physician should always act in best interest of the patient.

F. Committed Mentally Ill. If a person is committed for psychiatric reasons, certain conditions are also present.

   1. Must have treatment available.

   2. The patient can refuse treatment.

3. The patient can require a jury trial to determine "sanity."

4. The patient retains competence for conducting business transactions, marriage, divorce, voting, driving, etc.

5. Sanity and competence are legal terms, not psychiatric diagnosis.

6. Restrictions on patient:

   a. Civil liberty to come and go.

   b. Emergency detention can be effected by M.D. or law enforcement for 48 hours pending a hearing.

   c. M.D. can detain; a judge can commit.

   d. **With children, M.D. cannot detain;** only parents or juvenile courts can do so.

      (1) only for imminent danger to self or others;

      (2) can't care for self;

      (3) parents have no control over dangerous behavior (fire-setting).

G. <u>If a patient refuses treatment</u>:

   1. If life threatening can treat to save the life.

   2. If not life threatening one must determine if they have the ability to make decisions; e.g., do they have a psychotic level disorder (e.g., delirium, Brief Reactive Psychosis, etc.).

   3. Physician can detain against the patient's will if they are a danger to self or others. Can't treat against the patient's will unless they are a danger to self or others.

   4. If can't detain and the patient wants to leave, try to get they to sign a document that they are leaving Against Medical Advice (AMA). If they won't sign, carefully document all actions in the patient's records. "If it's not written down, it didn't happen."

H. <u>Privileged Communication</u>: Generally the following hold.

1. If the person is a threat to self or others you can break confidentiality and notify the victim, police. Helps legally if you have told the patient in advance of these potentials.

2. Police can't do anything until the patient does something, unless it is the President, a Senator, the Pope, etc. Otherwise need a release of information.

3. Real controversy today regarding legal issues and suicide/homicide and breaking confidentiality.

I. <u>Duty to Warn</u>

1. Due to the landmark Tarasoff Decision by the California courts, psychotherapists are required to report intents not fantasies of homicide or suicide.

2. Also includes the duty to warn to protect others if the person is in a publicly responsible position; and, their impairment could have disastrous effects on other e.g., an actively alcoholic school bus driver.

CHAPTER 15

PSYCHIATRIC EMERGENCIES

I. VIOLENCE AND AGGRESSION

A. <u>General issues of Psychiatrist involvement in violence.</u>

1. Sometimes asked to help intervene in the acute condition, e.g., hostage taking, poised on the edge of suicide.

2. Sometimes must intervene with an Emergency Order of Detention (EOD) if the patient is a danger to self and/or others.

3. Sometimes asked to determine the mental condition of the person who has e.g., committed a rape; particularly if the individual is a recidivist and/or if the person's behavior suggests he may have been under the influence of an active psychotic process at the time of the event.

4. Often asked to see the victim to assist in the rehabilitation after the event has occurred.

B. <u>The Acutely Violent Person</u>

1. Psychiatric assistance is often requested in the situation where the violent person is threatening harm to another.

   a. Hostage for personal gains.

   b. Expression of an acute psychotic condition: e.g., listening to auditory hallucination.

   c. Toxic condition

      (1) Delirium secondary to infection, etc..

      (2) Recreational drug use which has become an untoward event ("bad trip").

2. Management is dependent upon the etiologic condition.

   a. In hostage situations there is little the general psychiatrist can do. This is a legal, political, law enforcement situation.

   b. If the person is acutely psychotic and hallucinating, often the psychiatrist can present as a non-threatening medical "friend" who is there to help the person, particularly if the psychiatrist had previous positive contact with the patient.

May need to effect an emergency hospitalization.

c. In the toxic conditions, sometimes the person must be subdued in a humane manner (i.e., if the person has an infectious encephalitis); or in the situation with recreational drug toxicity, it may be a matter of keeping the person engaged (biding time) while the drugs are metabolized from the body.

C. Rape

1. **General background on rape** (exclusive of prison)

   a. 3.5% - 10% are reported. One out of ten women will be raped at some time in their lives (Government surveys and predictions).

   b. It is a crime of violence, not of sexual passion.

      (1) for power

      (2) for control

      (3) for revenge against:

         (a) mistreating mother

         (b) rejection from other women

   c. Rooted in emotional immaturity.

      (1) sexually naive

      (2) very conservative sexual attitudes

      (3) "Typical Rapist"

         (a) 15-19 years old

         (b) in the summer not the winter

         (c) 50% in the victim's home

         (d) rapist is usually poor

         (e) 3/4 were sexually abused as children

         (f) 50% of rapist are known to some degree by the victim.

(4)   There is no known standard response to a rapist that will leave the woman unharmed. This point is important in the psychological rehabilitation of the victim.

2. **Treatment for the victim of rape:**

   a. It takes women from 6 months to 6 years to recover from the experience.

   b. Focus is on helping the person rid self of the guilt.

   c. Couples therapy to help the non-raped spouse overcome the belief that the significant other is now "damaged merchandise."

3. **Treatment for the rapist:**

   a. <u>Counterconditioning</u>

      (1)   Forced masturbation, e.g., for one hour, with rape fantasies until the penis becomes extremely sore.

      (2)   Let the person fantasize but change the ending to a terrible consequence. E.g., at the point in the fantasy that penetration is made and thrusting is begun, insert into the fantasy that there is a razor blade in the vagina and each time a trust occurs there is slashing of the head of the penis.

   b. Force the rapist to view films of the response of the victim, both short term and long term.

   c. <u>Drugs</u>: Depro-Provera. Leads to a decrease in testosterone levels and provides a chemical castration.

D. <u>Spouse Battering</u>

   1. **Statistics**

      a. These are very unreliable and represent the minimal amount that actually goes on.

      b. 4% of women are victims of beatings by their partners each year.

      c. A slightly higher percent of men are beaten by their partners each year. However, due to differential strength the men do not get hurt as badly; and, they do not tend to report it to police or emergency room personnel.

2. **The Male Beater:**

   a. Beaten as a child

   b. Episode is like a temper tantrum of the child.

   c. Insecure: Female is the emotional glue that holds them together.

   d. Trying to make the female closer by controlling her physically.

   e. Charming/narcissist.

   f. Believes the woman is at fault.

      (1) Feels and believes that the woman did not live up to expectations.

      (2) Sees violence as an act of communication.

3. **The female who is beaten:**

   a. Often has grown up in violence and accepts it as a pitiful form of caring. She is often afraid of the world and wants protection from the world, even by the man who beats her.

   b. 25% of female suicide attempts are preceded by a prior history of battering.

   c. Often from a home where she saw mother beaten and accepts it as her role.

   d. There is __NO__ support for the theory that she derives masochistic pleasure from the beating.

   e. Culturally women are conditioned to hold the family together at all costs. Also, some cultures and subcultures teach that it is O.K. to beat your wife (1/6 women and 1/4 men endorse this concept).

   f. The women believe their husbands have chronic emotional problems and are therefore __NOT RESPONSIBLE__.

   g. The woman feels the beatings are coercive, hostile and intended to cause injury.

h. Ann Page (a researcher in the area) believes the woman stays with the man because of fear of loneliness and nonsupport. Probably the latter is the most important.

4. **The Cycle:** (Reference: Walker, L. _Battered Women_)

   a. PHASE I: Initial tension building phase: verbal abuse, minor violence (e.g., throws a plate of food across the room or at the woman). The woman still feels like she has some control, avoids certain situations and topics and keeps the children away from him. This phase can last weeks, months, or years.

   b. PHASE II: Phase I episodes become more frequent and finally erupts in an episode of violence of 2-24 hours.

      (1) No matter what the woman does she cannot stop the man's actions. If the police are called it's during this phase of beating; however, many do not call because they don't feel anything can protect them from the violence and it might make it worse.

      (2) If the woman does not take action on the very first time that this occurs, the male assumes that she agrees with the contract, that these are the roles, and it will continue.

   c. PHASE III

      (1) After the outburst the man is usually calm, loving, kind, contrite, charming, etc.

      (2) Promises to change and convinces her that he is the man she fell in love with. This is the reinforcement for staying in the marriage.

      (3) In actuality, this third part of the cycle is an attempt to control the woman by sending roses, etc.

5. **Treatment of the victim**

   a. Support for removing self from the abusive situation.

   b. If both persons are interested, couples therapy to deal with the predisposing, current and future structure of the relationship.

    c. If the couple breakup, treatment for the wife to help her cope with the psychic trauma of the battering.

E. Child Abuse

1. Background Data

    a. 90% of inmates claim they were abused children.

    b. Low socioeconomic status gets reported; and, high socioeconomic status gets treated.

    c. The best National survey to date reported that 3.6% of children are at risk of serious injury each year.

2. **Definition**

    a. Physical Abuse: e.g., beating, scalding with hot water, burning with cigarettes, etc.

    b. Sexual Abuse: e.g., fondling, coerced oral sex, oral/anal/vaginal penetration, etc.

    c. Neglect: e.g., poor nutrition, inadequate clothing for the weather, etc.

3. **Psychiatric Model:** A psychiatric model of "sick" parents does not work to explain the issue of child abuse.

4. **Social Interactional Model:** (Parke, R.D. in _Child Abuse Prediction_. Editor, Starr, R.H.; Ballenjar Publishing Co., Cambridge, Mass., 1980).

When emotions and conditions push parents to the breaking point, emotions are often unleashed in the form of mental and physical abuse. Children being the last remaining subject of domination are often the scapegoats for frustration and powerlessness.

    a. The culture

        (1) In cultures where children's rights are ignored there is a high rate of child abuse.

        (2) The level of violence in society appears to be reflected in the amount of violence in the family.

        (3) There is a high positive correlation between the cultural approval of physical punishment as

a child rearing tactic and physical child abuse.

(4) In cultures where more cognitive types of disciplinary techniques are used there is less child abuse.

b. The Community

(1) The Community's attitude towards children's rights, which may or may not be the same as the culture's.

(2) The Community's attitudes and values concerning the appropriateness of different kinds of child rearing tactics, which again may be the same or different than the predominant culture.

(3) The availability of informal support systems: E.g., the shift from extended family living arrangements to nuclear family living arrangements. This also includes neighborhood or community based organizations r groups. Where the neighborhood is a close nit and integrated one, child abuse decreases.

(4) Formal support systems, e.g., health care facilities, counseling services, employment agencies, etc..

(5) Abuse specific support systems, e.g., systems to reduce stress on families, providing education for child rearing.

c. The Family

(1) 90% of abusive parents were abused.

(2) Females abuse at a higher rate than males do probably because they spend more time with children; and single mothers have higher rates probably aggravated by economic circumstances.

(3) Male child abusers tend to be fathers, step-fathers or boyfriends.

(4) There is a high positive correlation between unemployment and physical abuse, probably reflecting the fact that stress over money leads to a "short temper."

(5)   Abusive parents tend to fall in three clusters:

    (a)   Parents with continual and pervasive hostility and aggression which is sometimes focused and sometimes directed at the world in general.

    (b)   Parents with characteristics of rigidity, compulsiveness, lack of warmth, lack of reasonableness and minimal pliability in thinking and belief. Considerable rejection of the child is noted. <u>They feel self-righteous and defend their right to act as they did in abusing their child.</u>

    (c)   Strong feelings of passivity and dependence. Many are unassuming, reticent and very unaggressive. <u>Often competed with the child for the love and attention of their spouse</u>. Generally depressed, moody, unresponsive and unhappy. They are immature people.

(6)   The parents as a general rule are not emotionally available to the abused child. Child abuse can be looked upon as a very severe case of nonbonding with the indicated child.

(7)   The families tend to be socially isolated.

    (a)   The family is larger than average size.

    (b)   Positive correlation with spouse abuse.

d. <u>The Child</u>:

The child contributes due to attributes which are no fault of their own, but which make them <u>different</u>.

(1)   Common Characteristics are: Abnormal pregnancy, difficult delivery, neonatal separation, other separations in the first six months, illness of the child in the first year of life, unwanted, unusually brilliant or retarded, physically handicapped, and the child is perceived as "ugly."

(2)   Personality characteristics of children who are abused (<u>no data to indicate whether these are cause or effect issues</u>) include: From the most to least frequent: Impaired capacity to enjoy

life, psychiatric symptoms (enuresis, temper
tantrums, headaches, bizarre behavior), low
self-esteem, school learning problems,
withdrawal, opposition, hyper-vigilance,
compulsivity, pseudo-mature behavior. These
variables are derived from multiple different
studies.

If one compares multiple different studies the
most common variables that show up between the
studies are: Hyper-vigilance, anxiety, and low
self-esteem.

e. The Abuse Event: The general paradigm that is seen
is:

(1)   In a child who is predisposed to becoming an
abused child by variables that the child has
which are different;

(2)   In a family which is socially isolated under
certain kinds of stresses like financial
issues;

(3)   In a community which is fragmented and provides
minimal social support;

(4)   In a culture which condones physical punishment
as the mechanism for child discipline and does
not respect the rights of children;

(5)   There will come a triggering event such as no
money from unemployment, the child crying
because it is hungry, other children in the
family also adding stress, the parents being
angry and then taking the physical punishment
disciplinary measures in a situation of
uncontrolled anger.

Frequently the battering of children occurs
when there is a quarrel between caretakers and
in approximately 50% of the cases the
caretakers are under the influence of alcohol.
One can also add to this that in some instances
the caretakers are mentally or emotionally
disturbed and the mounting stress precipitates
the event.

When the child abuse is sexual abuse the abuser
usually sees themselves as "loving" the child.
They do not perceive their behavior as being
"abnormal." It should be noted that incest is

reported in families with children being
victims under the age of two years old.

5. **THE MAJOR IMPORTANT ISSUE IS TO BELIEVE THE CHILD IF THEY MAKE A CLAIM.**

   a. **Children this age rarely lie about such a behavior in the adult person who is supervising them.**

   b. **However, be cautious about the child who has been "coached" to "get at" the other parent. E.g., child uses inappropriate, technical words, e.g., "He inserted his penis into my vagina." Reported by a four year old.**

6. **Treatment of the abused child**

   a. Usually requires extended and very supportive psychotherapy.

   b. Must help the child overcome the feeling of having deserved the abuse.

   c. If is sexual abuse, the child (or adult who was abused as a child) must deal with the betrayal of trust involved in the abuse by a caretaker.

II. **SUICIDE**

   A. General issues in suicide.

   1. **Definition:** The intentional termination of one's own life. A continuum from covert to overt action.

      Sometimes this is done in anger as emotional blackmail. Sometimes the individual is in extreme and unremitting discomfort and chooses to terminate their existence. Herodotus (c. 485 B.C.-425 B.C.): "When life is so burdensome, death has become for man a sought-after refuge."

   2. One of the 10 leading causes of death in America. About 30,000 each year (this is a minimal estimate).

   3. Studies of those who complete suicide show that their life circumstances were no worse than others. They had many alternatives; however, they didn't see the alternatives.

B. Primary Motivations

1. **Anger:** Overt motivation is to change others' attitudes and behaviors. "I'LL SHOW YOU, YOU SON-OF-A-BITCH. YOU'LL MISS ME WHEN I'M GONE." That is, there is an attempt to punish loved ones. Often this is a cry for help.

2. If appropriate anger and aggression can't be expressed, displaced, or scapegoated, it may be turned inward on self. This can lead to sadness and grief with a sense of futility.

3. Lack of future orientation or disastrous future: pain, mental illness, economic problems, a dreaded disease, etc.

4. These can end in depression which most Americans ignore in self and others. Studies of medical personnel in outpatient clinics indicate they miss approximately 85% of the depression in patients.

5. **The Triad**

   a. Worthlessness: "I have no value to anyone. No one calls me, no one invites me to places, and there is no one who loves me."

   b. Hopelessness: "Things will never change."

   c. Helplessness: "There is nothing I can do to change this situation."

   Coupled with psychological and physical exhaustion: "I just can't go on."

6. Many report a sense of great relief with the act itself.

C. Secondary motivations:

1. To provide a sense of power and control to bolster feelings of inadequacy. "I have final control over this life of mine."

2. Loss of status or self esteem. Self esteem based on success, recognition and achievement. High producers who experience minor setbacks perceive more devastation. In the great depression of the 1920's it was the Wall Street persons and bankers who were jumping out of windows, not the farmers and laborers.

3. Join a deceased one. An expression of love. An avoidance of "going on" without the lost one.

4. Avoid becoming a problem. Very frequent with the elderly.

5. Seek martyrdom. The "Jonestown" mass suicide.

D. Attempters vs. Completers

1. Attempters: younger, female, impulsive and ambivalent, neurotic, personality disorders, chemically dependent, situational disorders.

2. Completers: Older, male, lethal techniques, major affective disorders (NOTE: 40-70% of completers have a diagnosis of depression.), alcoholism (7-21% of alcoholics commit suicide), addicted, schizophrenic.

3. Serious persons who survived: Poised between life and death with intense ambivalence about dying. Can't make plans (e.g., lunch date) because they expect to be dead. Felt/believed suicide was inevitable. What they wanted was a change in their life.

E. Biochemistry

1. 5-HIAA (a serotonin metabolite): Low levels have been found in the spinal fluid of depressed people and people who have killed themselves.

2. It is also low in the spinal fluid of persons who show antisocial, aggressive or impulsive personality traits.

3. It may be that 5-HIAA has to do with regulation of violence, aggression and impulsiveness.

F. Immediate Management

1. If you suspect ... ASK! It does not offend the person but rather gives them the awareness that at least one other person in the world cares about them.

2. Don't challenge or try to use shock methods: E.g., "Well just go ahead and do it". In the Emergency Room punishment doesn't help. E.g., don't pass the nasogastric tube with no lubrication on it.

3. If it is a telephone call:

    a. Reassure that you are there: Not 24 hours a day but you are there. (This is also true of non-telephone contacts.)

    b. Talk and get them to talk. Dont allow long silences.

4. Active listening

    a. Assess level of severity (e.g., thoughts, plans, impulses, actions).

    b. Evaluate plans.

5. Get the person oriented to the future: e.g., plan for the next 24 hours.

6. Cover the last 24 hours to try to find the trigger.

7. Get a "no suicide contract" or hospitalize the person.

8. DON'T MAKE A CONFIDENTIAL CONTRACT WITH THE PERSON.

9. Be ready to take charge: call family, call police, commit, etc.

G. Long Term Management

1. Make the environment safe: e.g., remove guns, medications, etc.

2. Seek professional help. Get a consultation with appropriate persons.

3. Beware of elevated moods and quick recoveries. Quick recoveries tend to lead to future suicides.

Demographic Factors in Suicide

	High Risk	Low Risk
Age	45 - Over	45 - Under

Risk steadily increases with age:

A. Children: Suicide is rare, but approximately 12,000 per year are hospitalized for self destructive acts: e.g., stabbing, cutting, scalding , burning, OD, jumping from high places.

B. Adolescents: Third most common cause of death (accidents and homicides are #'s 1&2). In those that try or succeed, there is a high incidence of parental abuse or neglect.

C. College students: Second most common cause. Accidents are first. Most on the basis of loneliness.

D. Elderly: are 10-16% of the population but commit 23-25% of the suicides.

   1. There are major issues of illness and independence for the elderly.
   2. They are experiencing all types of losses.
   3. They may be in abusive family situations of drugs and violence; however, they have no alternatives but to remain in the situation.

	High Risk	Low Risk
Sex	Male	Female

Males represent 3/4 of all suicides.

	High Risk	Low Risk
Race	White	Non-White

Of the 3/4 who are males, 70% are white. However, black male suicide rate is increasing.

	High Risk	Low Risk
Religious preference	Protestant	Catholic

	High Risk	Low Risk
Marital Status	Separated, divorced, widowed	Single, married

	High Risk	Low Risk
Socio-Economic-Status	High and Middle	Lower

Physicians: 1.5-2.0 times general population

However, if one controls for the social class, physicians do not have any higher rate of suicide than their colleagues.

	High Risk	Low Risk
Employment	Unemployed	Employed

Unemployment tends to undermine the personal/familial stability and trigger other problems.

	High Risk	Low Risk
Living Arrangements	Alone	With Others

There may be a general point here of the person who is isolated or is beginning to isolate themself.

	High Risk	Low Risk
Health	Poor	Good

	High Risk	Low Risk
Daily Routine	Changed (e.g., running, church attendance)	No Change

Most put order to their lives immediately prior to the suicide as if they are going on a trip. They set things in order first.

	High Risk	Low Risk
Mental Condition	Nervous/Mental Disorder (including alcoholism)	Normal

Almost 95% of patients who commit or attempt suicide have a diagnosed mental illness. Depression is the most common by far.

Alcohol: is a depressant drug and will exacerbate a depression. Also, the drug takes away the "thou shalt not's."

Avoid the exacerbations of psychiatric illnesses.

Psychotic process fulfillment: Voices telling the person to kill self.

Tends to run in families. This may be a spurious correlation through the familial distribution of depression and alcoholism.

	High Risk	Low Risk
Disposition	Admitted to Psychiatric Center	Discharged to self or relative.

Most are undecided: they gamble that someone will find them. Usually a person is only suicidal for a relatively brief period of time.

People discharged from mental hospital - 34 times more likely than general population. This is probably on the basis that the more severe cases of depression are hospitalized; they begin to feel better, are discharged too soon, and now they have the concentration and energy to carry out the suicidal thoughts which are usually the last portion of a depression to be relieved.

Most occur within 3 months after "improvement" of major depressive episode.

Contact with physician: Usually have been in contact with the physician in the recent past (e.g., 6 months).

	High Risk	Low Risk
Suicide note	Yes	No

If no note has been left, usually there has been some suicidal talk: e.g., "You'd be better off without me."; "I've had it."

8/10 have given a warning of some type.

	High Risk	Low Risk
Previous attempt	Yes	No

	High Risk	Low Risk
Method	Hanging, firearms jumping, drowning	Cutting, gas CO_2-poison

More women are beginning to use guns which is a more certain method than drugs or gas.

If drugs are used, usually the classes of drugs involved are the sedative-hypnotics (e.g., sleeping preparations), antidepressants, and minor tranquilizers.

	High Risk	Low Risk
Potential Consequence of method	Likely fatal	Harmless

	High Risk	Low Risk
Police description of condition of patient	Unconscious/ semi-conscious	Normal, disturbed, drinking, ill

III. **CHILDHOOD AND ADOLESCENT EMERGENCIES**

A. Descriptions

1. **Life Threatening Emergencies**

   a. Suicide and/or Homicide: About 50% of child emergencies are for suicidal threats or behaviors. May be thought, plans or attempts. Always take the child seriously.

   b. Care-taker cannot control the violence or aggression of the child. 25% of referrals are for assaultive, destructive (e.g., fire setting), and violent behaviors. May be Conduct Disorders

   c. Severe Anorexia Nervosa

2. **Non-Life Threatening Emergencies**

   a. Severe anxiety-panic symptoms.

      (1) The child/adolescent or parenting figure experiencing a serious or painful medical illness

      (2) The household is very chaotic. E.g., parenting figures are fighting with each other; a parenting figure is acutely/chronically mentally ill, etc..

      (3) A wrongdoing by the child/adolescent is discovered or is about to be discovered. The child/adolescent fears humiliation or severe punishment.

      (4) Separation Anxiety (School Refusal): Interpersonal problems with peers or siblings; parenting figure has been recently ill.

   b. Acute Psychotic Event: e.g., Schizophrenia, Major Depressive Episode, postconcussion delirium.

   c. Runaway behaviors or threats

B. General Etiologies to Consider

1. Drug use with an untoward reaction: Stimulants, psychedelics, cannabis, alcohol, etc..

2. Serious family pathology: incest, child/adolescent beating, severe neglect of the child, family chronically

intoxicated, family is chronically violent with each other, etc..

3. Recent health problem for the child/adolescent, e.g., encephalitis, diabetes, severe burn with body scaring, etc..

4. Loss of a parenting figure: e.g., death, divorce, etc..

5. Family crisis event: e.g., someone else attempts suicide, a parenting figure or sibling has an acute psychotic episode.

6. Legal difficulties for the child/adolescent or family, e.g., bankruptcy, 5th DUI for the adolescent, placed under arrest, etc..

7. Environmental change: e.g., recent relocation of family either on a voluntary or involuntary basis.

C. <u>Treatments</u>

1. Insure safety of the child/adolescent. This may include hospitalization.

2. Attempt to determine the precipitating event(s).

3. If it is a expression of an underlying Psychiatric Disorder, treat the disorder.

4. Where there is an indicated family, involve them in the problem solving. Often will require seeing the entire family including sibs, etc..

5. Reintegrate the child into the feared situation as soon as possible (e.g., school refusal).